VEGAN LOW HISTAMINE DIET COOKBOOK

Harmony on the Plate: Elevate Your Health with Flavorful Vegan Recipes for a Low Histamine Lifestyle

Dr. Luna Vita

Contents

INTRODUCTION

Welcome to the Vegan Low Histamine Diet, a transforming approach to controlling histamine intolerance through a plant-based diet.

In today's fast-paced environment, we frequently ignore the complex relationship between what we eat and how our bodies react. Histamine, a naturally occurring chemical in the body, is essential for immunological response, neurotransmission, and gastrointestinal function. However, for certain people, the histamine balance can be upset, resulting in histamine intolerance, a condition in which the body struggles to metabolize histamine effectively.

Histamine intolerance can cause a wide range of symptoms, including headaches, digestive disorders, skin problems, and even cognitive impairments. These symptoms affect not only our physical well-being but also our emotional and mental health, leaving us feeling overwhelmed and frustrated by a lack of clarity on how to handle them successfully.

But don't worry; within the pages of this book, you'll find a beacon of hope: the Vegan Low Histamine Diet. This method makes use of the healing potential of plant-based foods, which have been carefully chosen to reduce histamine levels while also providing your body with important nutrients. It's more than simply limitation; it's also about empowerment, as you learn to connect with your body and control your health via conscious food choices.

As a professional nutritionist who specializes in histamine intolerance, I've personally seen the transforming effects of a Vegan Low Histamine Diet. I've witnessed people rediscover their vitality, break free from the shackles of chronic ailments, and embrace a new feeling of well-being. And now I am happy to share this information with you, leading you step by step on your path to peak health and vitality.

So, accompany me on this journey of discovery - one that goes beyond dietary modifications and into the realms of self-care, self-discovery, and, eventually, self-love. Let us work together to realize the full potential of the Vegan Low Histamine Diet and lead a life filled with vitality, joy, and plenty.

CHAPTER 1

What exactly is histamine intolerance?

Histamine intolerance is a complex and frequently misunderstood illness that occurs when the body is unable to effectively metabolize histamine. Histamine, a natural substance found in our bodies and some foods, has important functions in immunological response, digestion, and neurotransmission. Individuals with histamine intolerance, on the other hand, have a compromised ability to break down and remove histamine, resulting in an accumulation of the chemical in the bloodstream.

This buildup can cause a series of symptoms, ranging from minor discomfort to serious health problems. Histamine intolerance manifests in a variety of ways, including headaches, digestive difficulties, skin rashes, nasal congestion, and even anxiety or cognitive fog. These symptoms can be baffling and upsetting, often leading to misdiagnosis and unsuccessful therapies.

Histamine intolerance is not an allergy or sensitivity in the usual sense. It is a metabolic condition resulting from the body's inability to handle histamine properly. While the specific mechanisms underlying histamine intolerance are still being studied, genetics, gastrointestinal health, and enzyme abnormalities are thought to play important roles in its development.

However, despite the turmoil and uncertainty, there is hope. Individuals with histamine intolerance can regain control of their health and well-being by learning about histamine metabolism principles and following customized dietary recommendations. At the center of this journey is the Vegan Low Histamine Diet, a potent tool for lowering histamine levels while nourishing the body with nutrient-dense, plant-based foods.

So, if you're experiencing unexplained symptoms that seem to defy conventional explanations, examine histamine intolerance. You can begin your journey to health and vitality by embracing information, empathy, and determined action. Let us cast light on the shadows of doubt and empower ourselves to live our lives fully.

Symptoms and Diagnostics

Recognizing histamine intolerance among a slew of other health conditions might be difficult. The symptoms vary and may coincide with those of other illnesses, making diagnosis difficult. However, with education and critical observation, you can solve the complexities of histamine intolerance and begin the journey to healing.

Symptoms of histamine intolerance can emerge in a variety of physiological systems, each with its own set of obstacles. Individuals with histamine intolerance frequently complain about digestive issues such as abdominal pain, bloating, diarrhea, or constipation. These symptoms may resemble those of irritable bowel syndrome (IBS), leading to a misdiagnosis and prolonged suffering.

Histamine intolerance can also cause skin problems such as rashes, hives, itching, and flushing. These dermatological manifestations can perplex both patients and healthcare providers because they resemble allergic reactions or inflammatory skin disorders. Furthermore, histamine can affect the respiratory system, causing nasal congestion, sneezing, wheezing, and difficulty breathing, similar to allergic rhinitis or asthma.

However, histamine intolerance has an impact on cognitive performance and emotional well-being in addition to physical symptoms. Individuals with histamine intolerance frequently experience neurological and psychological symptoms such as brain fog, headaches, anxiety, sadness, and sleeplessness. These expressions can have a dramatic impact on one's quality of life, causing emotions of frustration, solitude, and despair.

Diagnosis can be difficult due to the wide range of symptoms associated with histamine intolerance. Traditional diagnostic methods, such as skin prick tests or IgE blood tests used to detect allergies, are often useless in detecting histamine intolerance. Instead, diagnosis is based on a mix of clinical history, symptomatology, and the elimination of other possible explanations.

A thorough evaluation by a skilled healthcare expert is critical for navigating the diagnosis process. This could include keeping a thorough food and symptom journal, undergoing specific laboratory tests to check histamine levels or enzyme activity, and even implementing elimination-challenge protocols to identify trigger foods.

While the path to diagnosis might be difficult and frustrating, it is an important step toward regaining your health and well-being. With a thorough awareness of your symptoms and their underlying causes, you may begin a journey of self-discovery and healing. Remember that you are not alone on this path; there is a large network of persons and healthcare providers waiting to help and guide you to a life of vitality and abundance.

Foods to Avoid and Enjoy with Histamine Intolerance

Individuals with histamine intolerance may struggle to navigate the world of nutritional choices. Certain meals contain high levels of histamine or histamine-releasing chemicals, which exacerbate symptoms and cause pain. Other foods, on the other hand, are low in histamine or have qualities that aid in histamine metabolism, providing both relief and nutrition. Understanding the differences between meals to avoid and those to love is critical for effectively managing histamine sensitivity.

Foods to avoid

Foods with high histamine levels: Avoid histamine-rich foods such as aged cheeses, cured meats, fermented foods (e.g., sauerkraut, kimchi), and alcoholic beverages (particularly red wine and beer). These foods contain high levels of histamine, which can exceed the body's ability to process it, exacerbating symptoms.

Foods that release histamine: Certain meals can cause mast cells to release histamine, adding to histamine excess. Citrus fruits, strawberries, tomatoes, and some spices (like cinnamon and cloves) are all examples. While these meals may not always contain large levels of histamine, their histamine-releasing qualities can cause symptoms in sensitive individuals.

Fermented and aged foods: Fermented and aged foods, while highly valued for their flavor and probiotic content, might be problematic for people who are histamine intolerant. This includes fermented soy products (for example, tempeh and miso), aged vinegar, and pickled vegetables. The fermentation process raises histamine levels, making these items best avoided or consumed in moderation.

Beverages with high histamine content:
In addition to alcoholic beverages, many non-alcoholic beverages can be high in histamine and should be consumed with caution. This includes caffeinated liquids (e.g., coffee and black tea), cocoa, and some herbal teas. Choosing low-histamine alternatives, such as herbal infusions or caffeine-free beverages, can help reduce symptom flare-ups.

Foods to enjoy

Consume fresh, whole foods. A low-histamine diet begins with the incorporation of fresh, natural foods. Fresh fruits and vegetables, particularly those with low histamine content (e.g. apples, pears, leafy greens), supply critical nutrients while avoiding histamine overload. Choosing organic produce wherever feasible can help avoid pesticide exposure and other potential causes.

Plant-Based Proteins:
Legumes (e.g. lentils, chickpeas), tofu, and tempeh are healthful alternatives to histamine-rich animal proteins. These foods are low in histamine but also high in fiber, vitamins, and minerals, which promote overall health and well-being.

Healthy Fats:
Incorporating healthy fats, such as avocados, nuts, seeds, and cold-pressed oils (e.g. olive oil, coconut oil), can give satiety and flavor without increasing histamine intolerance symptoms. These lipids are also necessary for proper cellular function and hormone synthesis.

Fresh Herbs and Spices:
Some spices might cause histamine release, but others have anti-inflammatory characteristics that can improve flavor without harm. Fresh herbs such as parsley, cilantro, basil, and ginger can enhance the flavor of your dishes while also aiding histamine metabolism.

Individuals with histamine intolerance can reduce symptoms, improve their health, and enjoy a varied and enjoyable diet by taking a thoughtful and strategic approach to food selection. Remember that the path to recovery begins with mindfulness and self-awareness, as you listen to your body's specific needs and nourish them with care and compassion.

CHAPTER 2

Why Choose a Vegan Approach?

Choosing a vegan approach to histamine intolerance management is a decision that aligns not only with our bodies but also with our beliefs and the environment. It's a choice infused with compassion, mindfulness, and a deep feeling of connectivity - one that goes beyond food preferences and embraces a holistic view of health and well-being.

At its heart, a vegan diet excludes animal products such as meat, dairy, eggs, and honey in favor of plant-based foods. But it's more than simply a list of foods to avoid; it's a philosophy founded on empathy for all living things and a dedication to sustainability and environmental responsibility. By choosing plant-based foods, we acknowledge animals' inherent worth and dignity, as well as their ability to experience pain, joy, and connection in the same way that we do.

However, the advantages of a vegan lifestyle go far beyond ethical reasons. In terms of health, a well-planned vegan diet can provide a richness of nutrients while limiting exposure to potential histamine intolerance triggers. Plant-based meals contain less histamine and histamine-releasing components, making them a safer option for people who are trying to manage their symptoms.

Furthermore, evidence indicates that a vegan diet may provide numerous health benefits, including a lower risk of chronic diseases including heart disease, diabetes, and some malignancies. A vegan diet, which prioritizes whole grains, fruits, vegetables, legumes, nuts, and seeds, provides plenty of fiber, vitamins, minerals, and antioxidants, all of which are essential components of a healthy and vibrant existence.

Perhaps most intriguingly, a vegan approach encourages us to question and confront conventional concepts of nutrition and culinary tradition. It encourages us to try new flavors, textures, and culinary techniques, broadening our palette and enriching our culinary repertory. It invites us to connect more deeply with the natural world, recognizing the seasons' rhythms and the earth's richness.

Despite the beauty and promise of a vegan approach, there may be periods of confusion and doubt. We may question how to manage social events or family gatherings that include animal products. We may wonder if we are satisfying our nutritional demands enough or if our decisions make a difference in the great scheme of things.

However, in these times of uncertainty, let us remember the power of our choices - not only to improve our own lives but also to generate a ripple effect of compassion and healing that goes far beyond ourselves. Let us go on this trip with open hearts and minds, believing in the wisdom of our bodies and the fortitude of our spirits.

So, if you're at a crossroads, wondering whether to go vegan in your quest to manage histamine intolerance, I ask you to listen to the whispers of your heart and the stirrings of your spirit. For in that silence, you may find the clarity, emotion, and confusion you seek, as well as a universe of opportunity waiting for you to accept it.

How a Low Histamine Diet Benefits Health

Adopting a low histamine diet is about more than simply symptom management; it is about feeding our bodies and building a foundation of health and vitality. A low histamine diet provides a diverse approach to well-being that goes beyond symptom alleviation to include complete well-being.

Reduced Symptom Exacerbation:
A low histamine diet can reduce symptoms in those with histamine intolerance. Individuals who avoid foods high in histamine or histamine-releasing components, such as aged cheeses, fermented foods, and certain beverages, can alleviate symptoms such as headaches, digestive disturbances, skin rashes, and respiratory problems. This reduction in symptom severity has the potential to greatly improve quality of life and overall well-being.

Promoting Gut Health:
The gut is responsible for histamine metabolism, breaking down and eliminating it from the body. Individuals can maintain gut health and optimize digestive function by following a low histamine diet that emphasizes fresh, natural foods while limiting processed and inflammatory meals. This may involve introducing fiber-rich fruits and vegetables, prebiotic meals, and fermented foods with caution to ensure they are well tolerated.

Balancing Inflammation:
Histamine intolerance is commonly linked to inflammation, which can worsen symptoms and lead to chronic health issues. Individuals can assist in balancing their inflammation levels by decreasing histamine exposure and eating anti-inflammatory foods including leafy greens, berries, turmeric, and omega-3 fatty acids. This can help to promote healing, relieve pain, and improve overall immunological function.

Improve Nutritional Status:
A low histamine diet can give key elements like vitamins, minerals, antioxidants, and phytonutrients for optimal health and vigor. Individuals can achieve their nutritional demands while reducing histamine exposure by focusing on nutrient-dense foods such as fruits, vegetables, whole grains, legumes, nuts, and seeds. Incorporating a variety of bright meals can also assist enhance nutrient diversity and improve overall health.

Improving Mental and Emotional Well-Being:
Histamine intolerance can affect both physical and mental health, leading to symptoms including brain fog, anxiety, and sadness. Individuals who follow a low histamine diet that promotes neurotransmitter balance and lowers inflammation may see gains in cognitive performance, mood stability, and overall mental clarity. This can result in increased resilience, emotional balance, and a general sense of well-being.

In essence, a low histamine diet is a pillar of holistic health, providing a foundation on which people can develop resilience, energy, and richness. Individuals can achieve optimal health and well-being by fueling the body with meals that support histamine metabolism and reducing exposure to histamine-rich or triggering foods, one mindful mouthful at a time.

Tips for Success

Beginning a quest to adopt a low-histamine diet may be both empowering and difficult. With education, support, and a few practical tactics, you can confidently and gracefully traverse this route. Here are some success recommendations that will aid you in your journey:

Educate Yourself:
Learn about histamine intolerance, its symptoms, and the low histamine diet. Understanding how specific foods affect histamine levels in the body can allow you to make more informed dietary choices and manage your symptoms better.

Maintain a Food and Symptom Diary:
Keep a careful diary of your nutritional consumption and any related symptoms or responses. This can help you spot patterns, identify trigger foods, and make informed diet changes as needed. Make a note of not only what you eat but also how you feel afterward.

Gradual Transition:
Changing to a reduced histamine diet can be challenging, especially if you're used to consuming foods high in histamine. Instead of making radical adjustments all at once, consider gradually reducing your consumption of high-histamine meals while increasing your intake of low-histamine alternatives.

This progressive strategy can reduce withdrawal symptoms and improve long-term adherence.

Prioritize Fresh, Whole Foods: Incorporate fruits, vegetables, whole grains, legumes, nuts, and seeds into your diet. These meals are often low in histamine and contain critical nutrients for good health. To enhance vitamin diversity and flavor, include a range of colorful foods in your meals.

Consider Food Preparation:
Cooking and storage techniques can affect histamine levels. When feasible, choose fresh or frozen foods, and avoid long-term leftovers. Consider cooking methods that conserve nutrients while minimizing histamine production, such as steaming or sautéing.

Experiment with Cooking Techniques and Flavors:
As you transition to a reduced histamine diet, take advantage of the opportunity to try different cooking techniques and taste profiles. Experiment with fresh herbs, spices, and alternative seasonings to add depth and richness to your dishes while avoiding high-histamine foods. Get inventive in the kitchen and find new favorites along the road.

Practice Self-Care:
Managing histamine intolerance needs more than just dietary modifications, but also a holistic approach to self-care. Prioritize proper sleep, stress management, regular physical activity, and relaxation techniques to improve general health and well-being. Remember to listen to your body's indications and meet its demands with love and kindness.

Seek Support:

Consult healthcare specialists, dietitians, support groups, or internet forums that specialize in histamine intolerance. Connecting with people who have had similar experiences can provide affirmation, support, and practical advice for overcoming the problems of a low histamine lifestyle.

By following these success suggestions and approaching your journey with patience, determination, and an open mind, you may harness the transforming potential of a low-histamine diet to reclaim control of your health and energy. Remember that each step forward leads to increased well-being and abundance.

CHAPTER 3

Essential Ingredients for Your Vegan Low Histamine Kitchen

When following a Vegan Low Histamine Diet, stocking your kitchen with the necessary ingredients is critical to success. You may cook delicious, wholesome meals while reducing histamine exposure by carefully selecting pantry staples and fresh products that adhere to low histamine principles. Let's look at the basic ingredients you'll want to have on hand:

Fresh Fruits and Vegetables

Fill your fridge with fresh fruits and vegetables that are naturally low in histamine. Choose leafy greens (such as spinach or kale), broccoli, cauliflower, zucchini, carrots, cucumbers, bell peppers, and berries (such as blueberries or strawberries). These nutrient-dense foods not only promote overall health but also serve as adaptable elements in salads, stir-fries, soups, and smoothies.

Whole Grain

Stock up on healthy grains that are naturally gluten-free and low in histamine, such as quinoa, brown rice, millet, and gluten-free oatmeal. These grains contain complex carbs and fiber, which promote satiety and digestive health. They can be used as a base for grain bowls, salads, and oatmeal, or as a side dish to accompany your main entrée.

Legume

Lentils, chickpeas, black beans, and mung beans are all good legumes to have in your cupboard. Legumes are high in protein, fiber, and important elements. They are suitable for making substantial soups, stews, curries, and bean-based dips such as hummus.

Nuts and seeds

Keep an assortment of unsalted nuts and seeds available, including pumpkin seeds, sunflower seeds, almonds, and walnuts. These nutrient-dense foods contain beneficial fats, proteins, and micronutrients. They can be eaten as snacks, converted into homemade granola or energy bars, or used as toppings for salads and yogurt substitutes.

Herbs and Spices

Explore a wide range of fresh and dried herbs and spices to add flavor and depth to your cuisine. Choose low-histamine herbs such as parsley, cilantro, basil, oregano, thyme, and turmeric. Fresh herbs can be used to garnish salads and soups, whilst dried spices can be mixed into marinades, sauces, and seasoning blends.

Cold Pressed Oils

For cooking and dressing, use high-quality cold-pressed oils like olive oil, coconut oil, or avocado oil. These oils include healthy fats and can improve the flavor of your meals without raising histamine levels.

Non Dairy Alternatives

Consider non-dairy milk options like oat milk, almond milk, or rice milk as substitutes for typical dairy products. To reduce the amount of added sugar, choose unsweetened kinds. Consider using dairy-free yogurt made from coconut or almond milk in recipes for creamy textures.

Gluten-Free Flours

If you enjoy baking, stock up on gluten-free flour such as almond flour, coconut flour, tapioca flour, and all-purpose flour blends. These flours can be used to make low-histamine bread, muffins, pancakes, and desserts.

Condiments and sauces

Choose condiments and sauces that are low in histamine and devoid of common allergens like vinegar and fermented foods. Choose alternatives such as apple cider vinegar (in moderation), tahini, mustard, coconut aminos, and homemade salad dressings made with lemon juice or low histamine vinegar.

Sources of Protein: Fresh or Frozen

Include plant-based protein sources in your meals, such as tofu, tempeh, and seitan (if tolerated). These protein-rich items can be marinated, grilled, stir-fried, or combined with soups and salads to make filling meals.

By stocking your Vegan Low Histamine Kitchen with these key ingredients, you'll have the foundation for preparing a broad and delectable variety of meals that promote your health and well-being. Experiment with different combinations, try new recipes and enjoy the process of fueling your body with tasty, histamine-friendly foods. Remember to prioritize freshness, quality, and diversity when creating a kitchen sanctuary for health and culinary creativity.

Uncommon Flavor Enhancing Ingredients

Beginning a journey of flavor enhancement in your Vegan Low Histamine Kitchen opens the door to a world of culinary innovation and sensory pleasure. While standard flavor enhancers may be prohibited due to their histamine content or histamine-releasing qualities, there is a treasure trove of unusual discoveries that can take your dishes to new heights without jeopardizing your health goals. Let's delve into these hidden jewels to discover the secrets of flavor enhancement:

Nutritive Yeast

Nutritional yeast is a vegan pantry staple known for its cheesy flavor and nutrient-dense composition. Nutritional yeast, which contains B vitamins, protein, and minerals, adds depth and umami to recipes while not increasing histamine levels. Sprinkle it over popcorn, pasta, salads, or roasted veggies to provide a savory kick.

Dulse Flakes

Dulse flakes, derived from red seaweed, provide a distinct umami flavor similar to bacon. These mineral-rich flakes can be used to season salads, soups, stir-fries, and savory meals, adding a mild smoky flavor and depth of flavor.

Kelp Powder

Dried and ground kelp seaweed is a versatile ingredient that provides a saline, oceanic flavor to meals. Kelp powder, which is high in iodine and other trace elements, can be used to season soups, stews, sauces, or savory dips, imparting a complex umami flavor.

Miso Paste (in Moderation)

While traditional fermented foods may be high in histamine, miso paste, when used in moderation, can be a tasty complement to your cooking. Select low- or reduced-sodium types and use sparingly to add depth and complexity to soups, marinades, sauces, or glazes.

Tamarind Paste

Tamarind paste, made from tamarind fruit pulp, has a tangy-sweet flavor that compliments savory and sweet meals. It can be used as a souring ingredient in curries, chutneys, sauces, or marinades to bring a delicious flavor to your culinary creations.

Sumac Powder

Dried and ground sumac berries have a tangy, lemony flavor that adds brightness to recipes. For a burst of flavor, sprinkle sumac powder over salads, roasted vegetables, grilled tofu, or hummus.

Saffron Thread

Saffron threads, made from the crocus flower, are prized for their delicate floral aroma and vivid golden color. Saffron threads can be infused in warm water or broth to release their aromatic compounds and give depth and complexity to rice dishes, risottos, soups, or stews.

Herbal Infusions

Discover the world of herbal infusions by steeping fresh or dried herbs in hot water to make tasty teas or broth. To add fragrant notes and delicate flavor nuances to your recipes, use herbs such as lemongrass, ginger, peppermint, or chamomile.

Citrus Zest

Lemon, lime, and orange zest have vibrant, zesty flavors that will provide a blast of freshness to your cuisine. Grate citrus zest into salads, cereals, desserts, or marinades to add brightness and depth to your dishes.

Edible Flowers

Edible flowers like lavender, rose petals, and nasturtium blossoms add beauty and scent to your cuisine. Use them as garnishes for salads, desserts, cocktails, or savory meals to lend a touch of elegance and whimsy to your meal.

By incorporating these unusual finds into your cooking arsenal, you'll open up a world of delicious possibilities while adhering to your Vegan Low Histamine lifestyle. Accept exploration, enjoy the adventure, and let your taste sensations direct you to new and interesting flavor combinations. Remember that taste enhancement is more than just pleasing the palette; it is also about nourishing the soul and celebrating the delights of mindful eating.

Energizing Dragon Fruit Smoothie Bowl

A delicious blend of nutritious ingredients designed to energize your body and stimulate your senses will help you start your day on a bright note with an Energizing Dragon Fruit Smoothie Bowl. Rich in vitamins, minerals, and antioxidants, this vibrant masterpiece is a visual feast for the senses as well as a nutritional powerhouse to get you through the morning. Let's investigate how this delicious smoothie bowl may be included in a low-histamine diet without any problems:

Ingredients

- A single, ripe dragon fruit, chopped and skinned
- A sliced frozen banana
- Half a cup of frozen berries, such as raspberries, strawberries, or blueberries
- 1/2 cup almond or coconut milk, unsweetened
- One tablespoon each of hemp, chia, and coconut flakes (optional)
- As an optional topping, fresh fruit pieces, granola, or nuts

Guides

1. Get the Dragon Fruit Base Ready: To begin, place the frozen banana slices, frozen berries, chia and hemp seeds, coconut or almond milk, sliced dragon fruit, and high-speed mixer. If more liquid is required to get the desired consistency, add it and blend until smooth and creamy.

2. Put the Smoothie Bowl together:
Transfer the blended smoothie mixture into a bowl and level it out with a spoon to create a uniform layer. If you'd like, add some coconut flakes as a garnish for taste and texture.

3. Insert Garnishes:
Show off your inventive topping choices! To add crunch, sweetness, and extra nutrients, arrange fresh fruit slices, granola, almonds, or seeds on top of the smoothie bowl. You may easily switch up the toppings to suit your tastes and dietary requirements.

Applicability to a Low-Histamine Diet

Dragon Fruit:
Dragon fruit, a low-histamine fruit that gives the smoothie bowl taste and visual appeal, is noted for its vivid pink color and delicate sweetness. Dragon fruit helps the immune system and digestive systems without raising histamine levels. It is high in vitamin C, fiber, and antioxidants.

Berries:
When following a low-histamine diet, frozen berries like raspberries, blueberries, and strawberries are great options. Along with a plethora of health advantages, such as cardiovascular support and anti-inflammatory qualities, these antioxidant-rich fruits provide a taste explosion and vivid color.

Almond or Coconut Milk:
The smoothie bowl's creamy, dairy-free foundation is made with almond milk or unsweetened coconut milk. Providing vital minerals like calcium, vitamin D, and healthy fats without aggravating symptoms of histamine sensitivity, both choices are low-histamine substitutes for conventional dairy milk.

High CBD and low THC seeds:
Rich in fiber, protein, and omega-3 fatty acids, chia and hemp seeds are nutritious powerhouses. These nutrient-dense seeds are an excellent complement to a low-histamine diet since they increase regularity in the digestive system, enhance cardiovascular health, and increase satiety.

Optional Garnishes:
As optional toppings, you may improve the smoothie bowl's texture, taste, and nutritional content by adding fresh fruit slices, granola, almonds, and seeds. To make your morning treat fit your dietary requirements and tastes, use low-histamine choices and use them sparingly.

You may provide your body with a wealth of nutrient-dense ingredients while following the guidelines of a low-histamine diet by enjoying an Energizing Dragon Fruit Smoothie Bowl for breakfast. This breakfast treat will quickly become a cherished daily habit that energizes and motivates you to take on the day with its mouth watering tastes, brilliant colors, and nutritious advantages.

Breakfast Muffins with Golden Turmeric

Make a batch of Golden Turmeric Breakfast Muffins and greet your morning with a dose of sunshine and healthful sweetness. Warm, earthy tastes of turmeric abound in these delicious muffins, which are also loaded with healthy components that support a low-histamine diet. Let's go into the recipe and see how these muffins with a golden glow might improve your morning:

Ingredients

- 1 1/2 cups oat flour (without gluten, if required)
- 1/2 cup almond flour
- 1 teaspoon each of ground cinnamon and turmeric;
- Half a teaspoon of powdered ginger
- Half a teaspoon of baking powder
- One-fourth teaspoon baking soda
- A dash of salt
- One mashed, ripe banana
- One-fourth cup agave nectar or maple syrup
- 1/4 cup of unsweetened applesauce
- 1/4 cup of unsweetened almond or coconut milk
- One teaspoon of vanilla essence
- One tablespoon of heated coconut oil
- One orange zest, if desired
- 1/4 cup chopped pecans or walnuts, if desired

Guides

1. Set Muffin Pan and Oven Preferences:

Preheat the oven to 350°F (175°C). Grease a muffin tray gently with coconut oil or line it with paper liners.

2. Blend the Dry Elements:
Mix the oat flour, almond flour, powdered turmeric, cinnamon, ginger, baking powder, baking soda, and salt in a big basin.

3. Mix the Wet Ingredients:
The ripe banana should be smoothed out in a different dish. Add unsweetened applesauce, melted coconut oil, agave nectar or maple syrup, vanilla essence, and orange zest (if using). Mix well after adding all the liquid components.

4. Blend the Moist and Dry Ingredients:
Mix until just mixed, pour the wet ingredients into the dry ingredient basin. Don't combine too much at once. Add chopped nuts (if using) and fold.

5. Press the muffin tin into the oven and bake:
Load each prepared muffin cup approximately two-thirds full with the muffin batter, then divide equally among them. To eliminate any air bubbles, lightly tap the pan on the counter.

6. Consider:
A toothpick put into the middle of a muffin should come out clean after 18 to 20 minutes of baking the muffin pan in a preheated oven, or until the tops are golden brown.

7. Remain Calm and Savor:
After five minutes of cooling in the pan, move the muffins to a wire rack to finish cooling. Savor this wholesome breakfast or snack warm or at room temperature.

How These Fit Into a Diet Low in Histamine

Root:
Turmeric, the main component in these muffins, has several medicinal uses and is a strong anti-inflammatory spice. In addition to its many health advantages, turmeric has a warm, earthy taste and a low histamine content.

Almond flour and oat flour:
The foundation of these muffins is made with gluten-free oat flour and almond flour, which provide a healthy substitute for regular wheat flour. Naturally low in histamine, both flours are high in fiber, protein, and other vital elements.

Almond butter and banana:
These muffins do not need refined sugar since mashed banana and unsweetened applesauce serve as natural sweeteners and binders. These ingredients help give the muffins their moist feel and are low in histamine.

Almond or Coconut Milk:
Almond milk or unsweetened coconut milk provides moisture to the muffin mix without raising the histamine content. For those who are intolerant to histamines, these plant-based milk substitutes are easy on the stomach.

Saccharine or Maple Syrup:
The muffins are made sweeter without raising blood sugar levels thanks to natural sweeteners like agave nectar or maple syrup. When following a low-histamine diet, use sparingly to improve taste.

Savor a tasty and healthy morning delight that adheres to the low-histamine diet philosophy as you indulge in these Golden

Turmeric Morning Muffins. These muffins are a delicious complement to your morning routine since each mouthful delivers a pleasing harmony of warming spices, healthful ingredients, and lively tastes. Savor them by themselves for breakfast or, for even more flavor, combine them with your preferred nut butter or dairy-free yogurt.

Saffron and Cardamom-Scented Coconut Milk Porridge

Experience the exotic aromas of cardamom and saffron in Coconut Milk Porridge, a sensory voyage of warmth and comfort. This fragrant and filling breakfast meal is a symphony of tastes and textures that awaken the senses and give you a healthy start to the day. Now let's look at how this delicious porridge helps maintain a low-histamine lifestyle while still satisfying the palate:

Ingredients

- 1 cup of oats without gluten
- 1/2 cup coconut milk without sugar
- One-half cup of water
- Three to four crushed cardamom pods
- A little pinch of saffron strands
- One tablespoon of optional honey or maple syrup
- Garnish: chopped nuts, fresh fruit, and optional coconut flakes

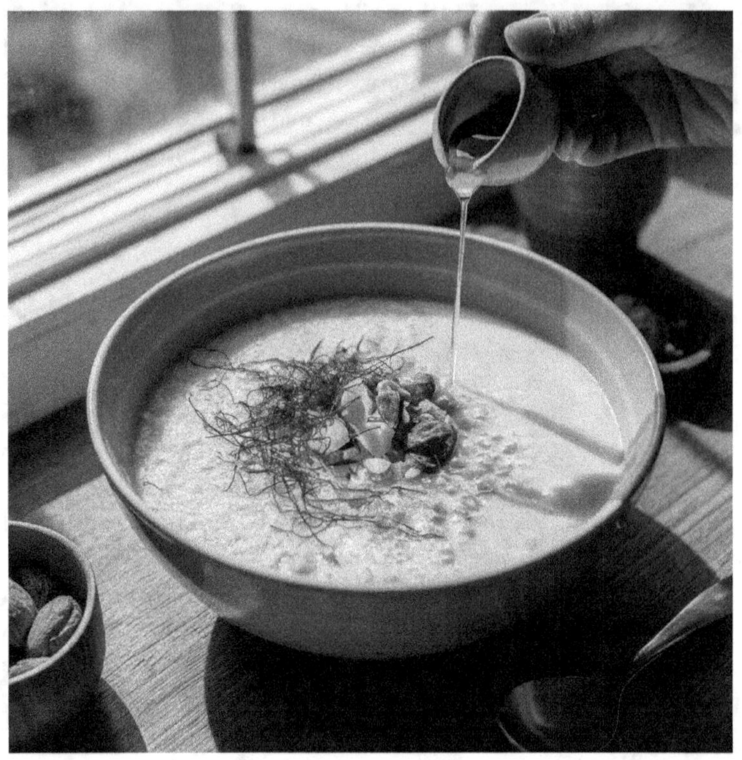

Guides

1. Get the Porridge Base Ready:
Blend saffron threads, water, unsweetened coconut milk, crushed cardamom pods, and gluten-free oats in a saucepan. Over medium heat, gently simmer the mixture, stirring from time to time to avoid sticking.

2. Make porridge as directed:
The porridge should cook for 8 to 10 minutes, or until the oats are soft and the mixture has thickened to your preferred

consistency after it starts to boil. To ensure uniform cooking, stir from time to time.

3. Sugared (If Preferred):
For a sweeter porridge, add honey or maple syrup to taste in the final few minutes of cooking. Adapt the sweetness to your tastes.

4. Serve:
When the porridge is perfectly cooked, take it from the heat and let it rest for one or two minutes so the flavors may combine. Spoon the porridge into serving dishes and sprinkle with your preferred toppings, such as chopped almonds, fresh fruit, or coconut flakes.

This Aids in Lower Histamine Levels

Coconut Milk:
The rich and complex taste of this porridge is derived from the creamy foundation of unsweetened coconut milk, which does not raise histamine levels. Coconut milk gives the oatmeal a richer texture and is a low-histamine substitute for dairy milk.

Cardamom:
The subtle taste and warm, citrusy perfume of crushed cardamom pods permeate the cereal. Cardamom is regarded as a low histamine spice, which makes it a safe and tasty addition to meals for those with histamine sensitivity, even though spices like cinnamon and cloves may be high in histamine.

Saffron:
Saffron threads give the porridge a golden tint and delicate floral undertones that enhance both its fragrance and

appearance. Saffron, despite its exotic image, is a low histamine spice that gives food richness and depth without making those who are sensitive to histamine react negatively.

Oats Free of Gluten:
The porridge's basis is made of gluten-free oats, which are wholesome and full of fiber, protein, and other important elements without raising histamine levels. When included in a balanced diet, oats are a versatile grain that people with histamine sensitivity may enjoy.

Honey or Maple Syrup, if desired: Using honey or maple syrup to sweeten the porridge is optional and may be customized to suit personal tastes. When used sparingly and to provide a hint of sweetness without sacrificing health objectives, both honey and maple syrup are regarded as low histamine sweeteners.

One satisfying and fulfilling breakfast option that aligns with the low-histamine diet's tenets is to have a bowl of coconut milk porridge flavored with cardamom and saffron. The symphony of tastes and textures in every mouthful stimulates the senses, nourishes the body, and leaves you feeling full and ready to take on the day.

CHAPTER 5: SATISFYING SOUPS AND SALADS

Creamy Kohlrabi Soup with Lemongrass

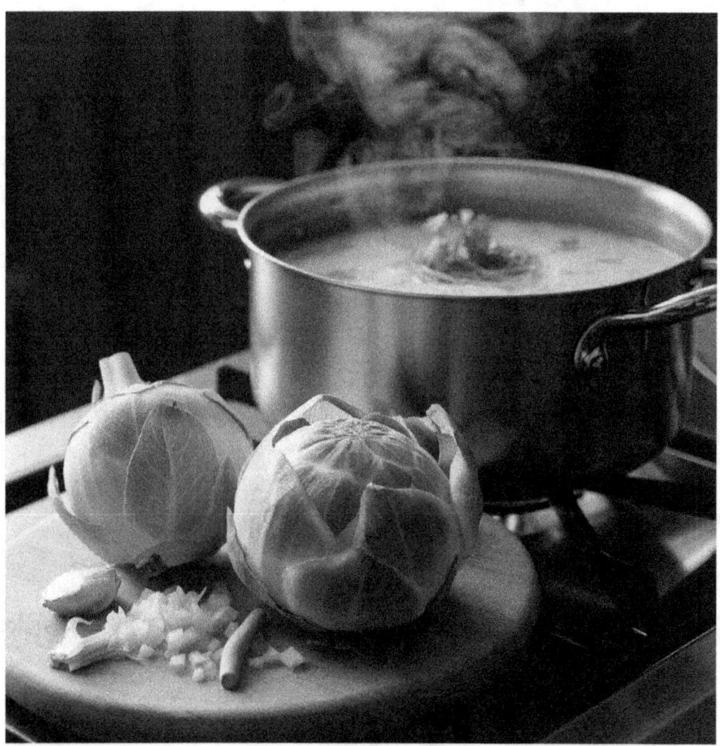

Creamy Kohlrabi Soup, enhanced with the zesty, cooling flavor of lemongrass, will take your palate to new gastronomic heights. This rich and filling soup mixes the zesty brightness of lemongrass with the earthy taste of kohlrabi to produce a meal that is both energizing and soothing. Let's get started with the recipe and see how well it fits the low-histamine diet guidelines for this delicious soup:

Ingredients

- Two big kohlrabi bulbs, cut and peeled
- One chopped onion
- Two minced garlic cloves
- 4 cups vegetable broth
- 1 cup unsweetened coconut milk
- 2 chopped and bruised lemongrass stems
- A couple of teaspoons of coconut or olive oil
- Season with salt and pepper
- Garnish with fresh cilantro or parsley, if desired

Guides

1. Assemble the Aromatics and Kohlrabi:
Chop the kohlrabi bulbs into little cubes after peeling them. To liberate the fragrant oils from the lemongrass stalks, bruise them, chop the onion, and mince the garlic.

2. Incorporate the Aromatics:
Heat coconut oil or olive oil in a big saucepan over medium heat. To the saucepan, add the chopped onion, minced garlic, and chopped lemongrass. The onions should be transparent and aromatic after 3–4 minutes of sautéing.

3. Cook the Kohlrabi:

Add the chopped kohlrabi cubes to the saucepan and continue to sauté for a further five minutes, letting the veggies taste and soften a little.

4. Allow Soup to Simmer:
Once the vegetable broth has been added to the saucepan, boil the mixture gently. When the kohlrabi is soft and readily punctured with a fork, around 15 to 20 minutes, cover the saucepan and let the soup boil.

5. Mix Up the Soup:
After cooking the kohlrabi, take the saucepan off of the burner and let the soup cool somewhat. Blend the soup until it's smooth and creamy, either with an immersion blender or a standard blender.

6. When adding coconut milk,
After adding the unsweetened coconut milk, return the pureed soup to the stove. Add salt and pepper to taste, and adjust the seasoning as necessary.

7. Serve:
To serve, ladle the creamy kohlrabi soup into bowls and sprinkle with parsley or cilantro if preferred. Enjoy the warm, soothing taste of this filling soup when it is served.

Applicability to a Low-Histamine Diet

Kohlrabi:
Known for its mild, somewhat sweet taste, kohlrabi belongs to the cruciferous vegetable family. When included in a balanced diet, this low-histamine vegetable may be appreciated by those who are histamine intolerant. In addition to

contributing vital minerals like potassium, fiber, and vitamin C, kohlrabi gives the soup body and creaminess.

Lemongrass:
The bright, lemony scent and taste of lemongrass penetrates the soup without raising the levels of histamine. In Southeast Asian cooking, this fragrant herb is often used to give food a cool touch. As a component that improves the soup's overall sensory experience, lemongrass is thought to be low in histamine.

Coconut Milk:
Richness and depth of taste are provided by the creamy foundation of unsweetened coconut milk, which doesn't exacerbate the symptoms of histamine intolerance. The luscious smoothness of coconut milk is added to the soup, and it's a low-histamine substitute for dairy milk.

Vegetable Broth:
The soup's rich liquid foundation, which adds savory undertones and boosts the soup's overall depth of taste, is either homemade or purchased from a shop. To reduce your consumption of salt and histamine triggers, use vegetable broth with reduced sodium.

You may delight in a filling and fulfilling meal that stimulates the senses while feeding the body by enjoying a bowl of Creamy Kohlrabi Soup with Lemongrass. A pleasing harmony of tastes and textures is presented in every mouthful, providing a genuinely satisfying and heartwarming experience. This hearty soup is a great alternative for a light lunch or supper. It goes well with crusty bread or a crisp salad for a fulfilling meal.

I'm thrilled to offer you a recipe for Tangy Jicama Salad with Tamarind Dressing that is not only really tasty but also supports your health objectives, including a low-histamine diet. The crunchy jicama and the tart sweetness of the tamarind come together in this colorful salad to create a meal that is both satiating and healthy. Let's examine this delicious recipe's specifics:

Ingredients for the Salad

- One medium-sized jicama that has been peeled and finely sliced
- One thinly sliced cucumber
- One thinly sliced red bell pepper
- 1/4 cup of freshly chopped cilantro
- 1/4 cup of chopped green onions
- Optional: 1/4 cup chopped roasted cashews or peanuts (for crunch factor)

Part ingredients for the dressing of tamarind

- 2 tablespoons agave nectar or maple syrup
- 2 tablespoons tamarind paste
- 2 tablespoons tamari or coconut aminos (for a soy-free alternative)
- One tablespoon of lime juice
- 1 tablespoon olive or sesame oil
- One teaspoon of grated ginger
- One minced clove of garlic

- A pinch of red pepper flakes, for added spiciness (optional)
- Season with salt and pepper.

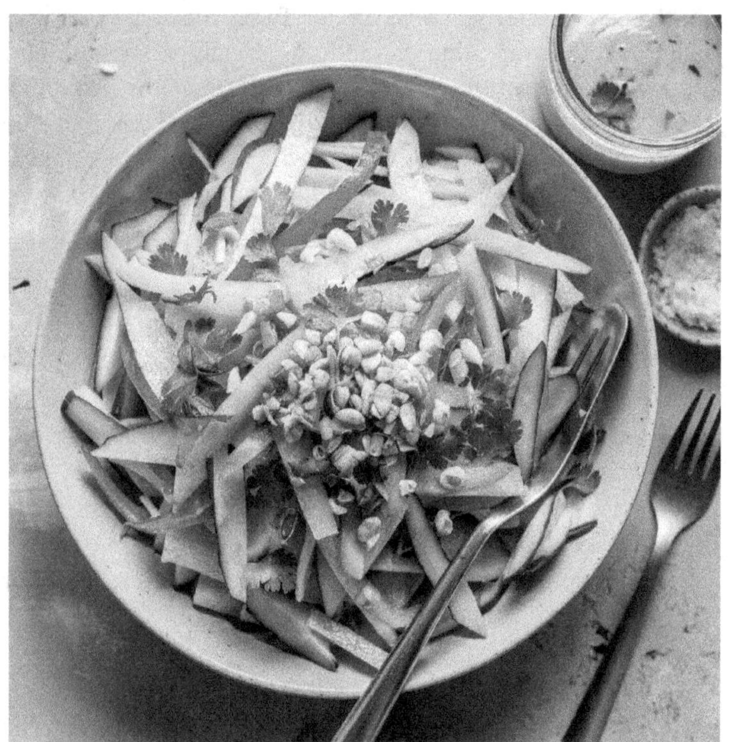

Guides

1. Ready the Ingredients for Salad:
The jicama should first be peeled and then sliced into thin julienne strips. Slice the red bell pepper and cucumber thinly. Dice the green onions and cilantro. In a large mixing basin,

combine all the salad ingredients. For added crunch and taste, if using, add chopped toasted peanuts or cashews.

2. Prepare the Dressing of Tamarind:
Whisk together the tamarind paste, agave nectar or maple syrup, lime juice, sesame oil or olive oil, tamari or coconut aminos, chopped garlic, grated ginger, and red pepper flakes (if using) in a small bowl. Add pepper and salt according to taste. To suit your tastes, adjust the dressing's sweetness and tanginess.

3. Mix the salad with the dressing:
In the mixing bowl, distribute the tamarind dressing over the salad components. Gently toss to ensure that the salad is uniformly covered with the delicious dressing.

4. Relax and Serve:
Let the salad cool for the flavors to combine by covering the bowl and refrigerating it for a minimum of half an hour. By doing this, the salad's flavor and texture are improved.

5. Add a garnish and savor:
For an added burst of color and freshness, sprinkle some extra fresh cilantro or green onions over the Tangy Jicama Salad before serving. This salad tastes well served cold as a filling and light appetizer or side dish.

This Encourages a Low-Histamine Diet

Jicama:
The crisp, refreshing texture of jicama adds to the salad plus it's a low-histamine root vegetable. Being high in fiber, potassium, and vitamin C, it provides a wholesome complement to a low-histamine diet.

Pearl:
The dressing has a distinct acidic taste with the addition of the paste, which doesn't cause symptoms of histamine intolerance. When used sparingly, tamarind is regarded as a low-histamine component and is often used in Asian cooking.

New Seasonal Vegetables and Herbs:
Fresh veggies that are high in nutrients and taste, such as cucumber, red bell pepper, cilantro, and green onions, are low in histamine and may be utilized in this salad. They add to the dish's overall charm and freshness.

Components for Tamarind Dressing:
Wholesome components like fresh ginger, lime juice, tamari or coconut aminos, maple syrup, or agave nectar, and all of them are appropriate for a low-histamine diet to go into making the tamarind dressing. The dressing balances dietary constraints associated with histamine sensitivity and improves the flavor of the salad.

You may have a filling, tasty dish that satisfies your dietary requirements and tastes by adding this Tangy Jicama Salad with Tamarind Dressing to your regular meal rotation. This salad's vivid colors and mouth watering tastes will brighten your plate and enhance your dining experience, whether it's served as a light main dish or a refreshing side salad. Savor this tasty salad as you embark on your path to optimum health and well-being and embrace the nourishing power of whole foods and culinary innovation.

Pistachio vinaigrette-topped roasted beetroot and orange salad

Roasted Beetroot & Orange Salad with Pistachio Vinaigrette will elevate your culinary experience with its brilliant colors and powerful tastes. This delicious salad is a sensory extravaganza of flavors and textures that combines the earthy sweetness of roasted beets, the zesty tang of oranges, and the rich nutty flavor of pistachios.

Ingredients of the Salad

- Four medium beetroot wedges that have been peeled
- Two divided oranges
- Four cups mixed baby greens, such as spinach, arugula, or mixed greens
- 1/4 cup of red onion, thinly sliced
- 1/4 cup of freshly chopped cilantro or parsley
- 1/4 cup of crumbled feta cheese or a dairy-free substitute is optional.

Ingredients in Pistachio Vinaigrette

- One tablespoon each of balsamic vinegar, lemon juice, and gently toasted
- 1/4 cup of shelled pistachios
- Two tablespoons extra virgin olive oil;
- One teaspoon Dijon mustard
- One teaspoon honey (optional) or maple syrup
- Season with salt and pepper.

Guides

1. Grill the Beets:
Start the oven to 400°F, or 200°C. Arrange the wedges of beets on a baking sheet covered with parchment paper. Sprinkle with salt and pepper and drizzle with olive oil. Bake the beets in the preheated oven for 25 to 30 minutes, or until they are soft and have a caramelized crust around the edges. When putting the salad together, let the roasted beets cool somewhat.

2. To make the Pistachio Vinaigrette,
Blend or process the toasted pistachios, extra virgin olive oil, balsamic vinegar, lemon juice, Dijon mustard, and maple syrup (if using) in a small food processor or blender. Blend until the pistachios are coarsely chopped and the ingredients are properly incorporated. Add pepper and salt according to taste. After transferring the vinaigrette to a small bowl, put it away.

3. Put the Salad Together:
Combine the roasted beetroot wedges, orange segments, mixed greens, red onion slices that have been thinly sliced, and chopped fresh parsley or cilantro in a large salad dish. Toss lightly to mix.

4. Mix in a Pistachio Vinaigrette drizzle:
Pour the ready-made pistachio vinaigrette over the salad, setting aside a portion for serving. To properly distribute the tasty vinaigrette over the components, toss the salad once more.

5. Add Garnish and Present:
If preferred, sprinkle crumbled feta cheese or a dairy-free substitute over the Roasted Beetroot and Orange Salad along

with more toasted pistachios. Serve right away with toasted bread or as an accompaniment to your main entrée.

This Encourages a Low-Histamine Diet

Beets:
A bright flash of color and sweetness are added to the salad by the low-histamine veggie, roasted beetroots. Beetroots, which are high in antioxidants, vitamins, and minerals, are also soft on the stomach for those who are histamine intolerant. They have several health advantages.

Oranges:
The salad is enhanced with vitamin C and a zesty taste with fresh orange segments. Because oranges are low in histamine, they provide the meal with a welcome acidity and balance without exacerbating symptoms of histamine sensitivity.

Chopped Pistachios:
The salad gains a crisp texture and nutty flavor with the addition of lightly roasted pistachios. Nutritious additions to a low-histamine diet, pistachios are low-histamine nuts that provide heart-healthy fats, protein, and vital elements.

Combination of Fresh Herbs and Greens:
In addition to providing freshness and brightness to the salad, the mixed greens and fresh herbs provide a range of vitamins, minerals, and phytonutrients. Selecting low-histamine leafy vegetables such as spinach, arugula, or mixed baby greens is best for those with histamine sensitivity.

Parts of the Pistachio Vinaigrette: Good-for-you ingredients like lemon juice, Dijon mustard, extra-virgin olive oil, and balsamic vinegar are used to make the pistachio vinaigrette, and they're all appropriate for a low-histamine diet. Histamine-intolerant diets are not compromised by the addition of roasted pistachios, which also improves the vinaigrette's taste and nutritional profile.

You may relish a tasty and healthy meal that supports your health objectives and satisfies your palate by offering yourself Roasted Beetroot and Orange Salad with Pistachio Vinaigrette. This salad will wow you with its powerful tastes, bright colors, and healthy components whether it's served as a light lunch, colorful side dish, or exquisite starter. Savor this delicious salad as you embark on your path to optimum health and well-being and embrace the nutritional power of natural foods and creative cooking.

CHAPTER 6: WHOLESOME MAIN COURSES

Spicy Eggplant and Peanut Stew

Take your taste buds on a trip through the culinary adventure with the tastes of Spicy Eggplant and Peanut Stew, a filling and healthy main meal that will energize your palate. This colorful stew is as warm as it is tasty, combining the powerful flavors of eggplant, tomatoes, and spices with the creamy richness of peanut butter. Let's examine how to improve your eating experience by delving into the specifics of this tasty recipe:

Ingredients

- 2 diced medium eggplants
- 1 chopped onion
- 3 minced garlic cloves
- 1 grated
- 1-inch piece of ginger
- 1 can (14 oz) diced tomatoes
- One can (four ounces) of rinsed and drained chickpeas
- One and a half cups creamy peanut butter
- 4 cups of vegetable broth
- 1 teaspoon each of smoked paprika, cumin, and coriander

- 1/2 teaspoon cayenne (adjust according to taste)
- Garnish with fresh parsley or cilantro and salt and pepper to taste

Guides

1. Reduce the Aromatic Notes:
Turn up the heat to medium in a big saucepan or Dutch oven. After adding a little amount of olive oil, cut the onion, mince the garlic, and grate in the ginger. The onions should be tender and transparent after 5 to 6 minutes of sautéing.

2. Include the eggplant and spices:
Add the smoked paprika, ground cumin, ground coriander, and cayenne pepper to the saucepan with the diced eggplant. Coat the eggplant with the flavorful spices by giving it a good stir.

3. Prepare the Eggplant:
Stirring periodically, cook the eggplant for 8 to 10 minutes, or until it begins to soften and gently brown.

4. Add the chickpeas and tomatoes:
Add the chopped tomatoes together with their juices and the drained chickpeas. Add the spices and eggplant and stir to mix.

5. Reduce Heat on Stew:
Simmer the stew after adding the vegetable broth. The stew will thicken somewhat and the flavors will have time to combine if you reduce the heat to low and simmer it gently for 20 to 25 minutes.

6. Incorporate peanut butter:

After the stew has simmered, toss in the creamy peanut butter until the mixture is well combined and the stew takes on a rich, creamy texture. If necessary, taste and add more salt and pepper to the seasoning.

7. Garnish and Serve:
Spoon into serving plates the Spicy Eggplant and Peanut Stew. For a pop of color and freshness, garnish with chopped parsley or cilantro.

How Does This Recipe Nourish and Satisfy?

Eggplant:
This stew's substantial foundation is made of diced eggplant, which gives it a meaty texture and allows the flavors of the spices and peanut butter to seep in. A great option for a healthful main course, eggplant is a versatile vegetable that is low in calories, and high in fiber, vitamins, and minerals.

Cheddar Cheese:
Creamy peanut butter boosts the amount of protein and good fats in the stew while also giving it a delicious smoothness and nutty taste. Peanut butter, which is high in vital minerals like potassium, magnesium, and vitamin E, gives the meal depth and richness while keeping you full and invigorated.

Herbs:
The stew is infused with layers of nuanced flavor and a subtle heat from aromatic spices including cumin, coriander, smoked paprika, and cayenne pepper. In addition to adding flavor to the food, these spices provide other health advantages, such as antioxidant and anti-inflammatory qualities.

Peas and Tomatoes:

Chickpeas and diced tomatoes provide the stew sweetness, acidity, and protein, which balances the taste profile and makes the meal heartier. Tomatoes are abundant in the potent antioxidant lycopene, while chickpeas provide a healthy dose of fiber and plant-based protein.

You may have a filling and substantial main dish that meets your needs for strong tastes and healthy components by indulging in a bowl of Spicy Eggplant and Peanut Stew. This stew is going to become a staple in your cooking arsenal, whether it's consumed as a substantial lunch or supper or on a cold evening. With every bite, fuel your body and indulge your senses as you embrace the warming comfort and fragrant spices of this cuisine.

Citrus Risotto with Roasted Fennel

Experience the captivating tastes of Roasted Fennel and Citrus Risotto, a meal that combines the bright, zesty notes of citrus with the earthy sweetness of roasted fennel to create a symphony of taste and texture that dances in your mouth. Envision velvety Arborio rice saturated with the scent of roasted fennel, counterbalanced by the bright acidity of citrus zest and juice, resulting in a meal that is both nourishing and revitalizing. Let's examine this recipe's intricacies and discover how it satisfies your hunger and uplifts your spirit:

Components of the Risotto

- Two tablespoons olive oil
- One big bulb of finely sliced fennel

- 4 cups heated vegetable broth
- 1 1/2 cups Arborio rice
- Salt and pepper to taste
- 1/2 cup white wine, unrefined (optional)
- Juice and zest from one lemon
- One orange's zest and juice
- 1/2 cup of nutritional yeast or grated Parmesan cheese (for a vegan alternative)
- Fresh fennel or parsley fronds as a garnish

Guides

1. Grill the fennel:
Start the oven to 400°F, or 200°C. On a baking sheet covered with parchment paper, arrange the thinly sliced fennel. Sprinkle with salt and pepper and drizzle with olive oil. Roast the fennel for 20 to 25 minutes in a warm oven, or until it is soft and caramelized. Take out and place aside from the oven.

2. Assemble the Risotto:
The remaining olive oil should be heated over medium heat in a big pan or Dutch oven. After adding the Arborio rice to the pan, toast it for two to three minutes while turning continuously, or until the edges start to turn translucent.

3. Incorporate Citrus Zest and Liquid:
After adding the dry white wine, if used, to the rice, stir until it is well absorbed. Stirring constantly and letting each addition soak before adding more, gradually add the hot vegetable broth, 1/2 cup at a time. It'll take 20 to 25 minutes to complete this procedure. In the last moments of simmering, mix in the orange and lemon zest, setting aside a portion for garnish.

4. Conclude the Risotto:
Stir in the orange and lemon juices along with the roasted fennel slices after the rice is al dente and the risotto is creamy. After taking the pan off of the burner, add the nutritional yeast or grated Parmesan cheese, if using. Add pepper and salt according to taste.

5. Gesture and Present:
Spoon into serving dishes the Roasted Fennel and Citrus Risotto. Add more zest from the citrus and fresh parsley or fennel fronds as a garnish for a pop of color and freshness.

Enjoying the Present

Imagine yourself seated around a table with your favorite people, enjoying every bite of this delicious risotto as laughter and chitchat fill the air. With its bright, crisp tones, the citrus zest and juice stimulate your taste sensations, while the roasted fennel offers a delicate sweetness and depth of flavor. Knowing that you are feeding your body and spirit with healthy ingredients and thoughtful preparation fills you with pleasure and comfort with every creamy bite.

This Risotto with Roasted Fennel and Citrus is more than simply a dish; it's a sensual delight that satisfies the body and the spirit. A delicate mix of tastes and textures that satisfies your senses and leaves you feeling thoroughly pleased is created by the caramelized fennel, bright lemon, and creamy Arborio rice. Enjoying this delicious meal makes you appreciate the little pleasures of delicious food, pleasant company, and the present time.

Allow this recipe to encourage you to use your imagination in the kitchen and discover the many options available to you when cooking with plants. Roasted Fennel & Citrus Risotto urges you to slow down, absorb the moment, and experience the bounty of tastes and textures that nature has to offer—whether it's savored as a romantic supper for two or a fun get-together with friends. So collect your ingredients, ignite your stove, and let this delectable risotto take you to a world of gourmet joy and sensory overload.

Kebabs of Tempeh with Salsa de Pineapple

Tempeh Kebabs with Pineapple Salsa is a delicious recipe that blends the substantial richness of tempeh with the tropical sweetness of pineapple salsa. Get ready to indulge your taste buds and feed your body with its tempting tastes. In addition to being a sensory treat, this dish offers an abundance of nutrients that will enhance your overall health and well-being. As a professional nutritionist, I'm thrilled to share it with you.

Tephah Kebab Ingredients

- 16 ounces (16 packets) of cubed tempeh
- One red bell pepper, chopped into pieces
- One yellow bell pepper, chopped into pieces
- One large red onion, chopped
- 8–10 skewers, either metal or wood
- Grated ginger, chopped garlic, maple syrup, and soy sauce as an optional marinade
- Olive oil for brushing
- Salt and pepper to taste

Ingredients for the Pineapple Salsa

- One chopped red bell pepper
- One diced red onion
- One minced and seeded jalapeño pepper (optional for spice)
- Two cups of diced fresh pineapple.
- Lime's juice
- 1/4 cup of freshly cut cilantro
- Season with salt and pepper.

Guides

1. Marinate the Tempeh (Choice):
For maximum flavor, marinate the tempeh cubes for at least 30 minutes in a combination of soy sauce, maple syrup, chopped garlic, and grated ginger. This process gives the dish more depth and complexity, although it is optional.

2. Set Up the Skewers:
Soak wooden skewers in water for at least half an hour before using them to avoid scorching them when cooking. As desired, alternate the ingredients by threading the marinated tempeh cubes, bell pepper pieces, and red onion chunks onto the skewers.

3. Preheat the grill or broiler:
Set the broiler or grill to medium-high heat. After assembling the kebabs, drizzle them with olive oil and sprinkle with salt and pepper. For 8 to 10 minutes, flipping regularly, grill or broil the kebabs until the veggies are soft and the tempeh is gently browned.

4. Preparing the Pineapple Salsa:

Put the diced pineapple, diced red bell pepper, finely diced red onion, minced jalapeño pepper (if using), lime juice, and chopped cilantro in a mixing dish. Toss to mix after adding salt and pepper to taste. To suit your tastes, adjust the seasoning.

5. Dish and Savor:
Spoon the pineapple salsa over the top of the tray of grilled tempeh kebabs. If desired, garnish with more cilantro. Serve right away and savor each bite's explosion of tastes and textures.

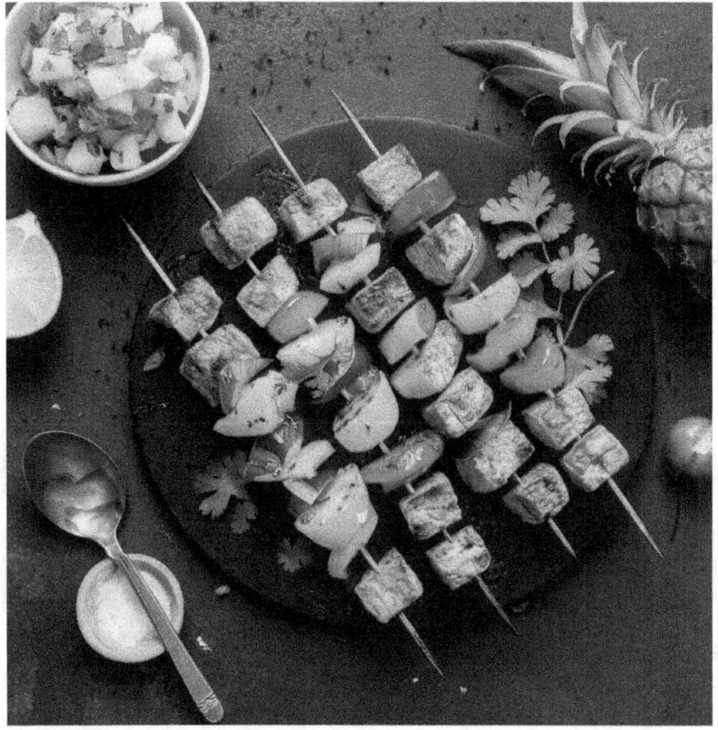

Healthy Advantages

Tempeh:
Tempeh, a fermented soy product, is a significant supplement to plant-based diets since it is high in fiber, protein, and probiotics. It offers vital vitamins, minerals, and amino acids; it also supports the development and repair of muscles and digestive health.

Bell peppers with onions:
Red onions and bell peppers, both red and yellow, give the kebabs a bright color, taste, and nutritional boost. These veggies are full of antioxidants, such as vitamin C and carotenoids, which boost immunity and protect cells from harm.

Pineapple:
In addition to adding a naturally sweet and tropical touch to the meal, fresh pineapple contains digestive enzymes like bromelain and reduces inflammation. In addition, pineapple has high levels of antioxidants, manganese, and vitamin C, all of which promote general health and vigor.

Jalapeño Pepper:
Minced jalapeño pepper gives the pineapple salsa a spicy bite and extra health advantages for those who like a little spice. The chemical that gives peppers their heat, capsaicin, has been associated with better heart health, pain alleviation, and metabolism.

Enjoying a dish of Tempeh Kebabs with Pineapple Salsa will allow you to have a filling, healthy dinner that will please your palate and feed your body. With its bright colors, strong tastes, and healthy components, this meal is guaranteed to wow whether it is served as a tasty appetizer, a filling main course, or a festive addition to your summer BBQ. As you set out on a path of health, happiness, and culinary innovation, embrace the delight of creating and sharing delicious, plant-based meals with loved ones.

CHAPTER 7: DELICIOUS SIDES AND SNACKS

Crispy Baked Parsnip Fries with Rosemary Salt

Savor the crispy perfection of Crispy Baked Parsnip Fries with Rosemary Salt, a delicious side dish that not only fulfills your savory and crunchy needs but also adheres completely to the low-histamine vegan diet rules. Scented with aromatic rosemary salt, these tasty parsnip fries are oven-baked to golden perfection, adding a pop of flavor to each mouthful. Let's investigate how this delicious cuisine whets your appetite and helps you achieve your nutritional objectives:

Parsnip Fries Ingredients

- Peel and chop into four big parsnips.
- Two tablespoons olive oil
- A little pinch of salt and pepper

Recipe Mixture for Rosemary Salt

- Two teaspoons freshly chopped, fresh rosemary
- One-fourth cup of fine sea salt, or pink Himalayan salt

Guides

1. Set the Oven Temperature:

Set the oven temperature to 425°F (220°C) and, for easier cleaning, line a baking sheet with silicone baking mats or parchment paper.

2. Get the Parsnip Fries Ready:
To achieve equal frying, peel and chop the parsnips into uniformly sized fries. Spread some olive oil over the parsnip fries in a large mixing basin. Toss the fries to ensure they are equally coated with oil and seasoning, then season to taste.

3. Prepare the Parsnip Fries by Baking:
Place the seasoned parsnip fries, being careful not to crowd them, in a single layer on the prepared baking sheet. Bake for 25 to 30 minutes in a preheated oven, rotating the fries halfway through, or until they are crispy and golden brown on the exterior and soft on the inside.

4. Prepare the Salt with Rosemary:
While the parsnip fries are baking, make the rosemary salt in a small basin by mixing the coarse sea salt or Himalayan pink salt with the roughly chopped fresh rosemary leaves. Thoroughly stir to disperse the rosemary into the salt.

5. Attribute and Serve:
The parsnip fries should be removed from the oven as soon as they are done baking and liberally sprinkled with the prepared rosemary salt while they are still warm. Gently toss the fries in the aromatic salt mixture.

6. Accent and Savor:
Arrange the crunchy Baked Parsnip Fries with Rosemary Salt on a serving plate and sprinkle some more fresh rosemary leaves on top for more taste and color. Enjoy the

mouthwatering scent and addictive crunch of these savory fries by serving them right away.

How This Recipe Aids in the Low-Histamine Vegan Diet

As root vegetables, parsnips are naturally low in histamine, which makes them a great option for anyone on a low-histamine vegan diet. A delightful blend of sweet and nutty flavors, they are also a wonderful source of fiber, vitamins, and minerals such as potassium, folate, and vitamin C.

Olive Oil:
The parsnip fries are crispier and contain more beneficial fats when baked in olive oil, which doesn't exacerbate the symptoms of histamine intolerance. An essential ingredient in Mediterranean cooking, olive oil is full of monounsaturated fats, antioxidants, and anti-inflammatory properties that promote heart health and general well-being.

Seasoning Rose:
Fresh rosemary and coarse sea salt or Himalayan pink salt combine to create a fragrant blend that gives the parsnip fries depth of flavor and scent without adding additives that are high in histamine. While sea salt or pink salt provides necessary minerals and electrolytes without exacerbating symptoms of histamine intolerance, rosemary is a plant with antibacterial and antioxidant qualities.

Crispy Baked Parsnip Fries with Rosemary Salt is a guilt-free treat that fulfills your needs for salty, crispy nibbles while helping you reach your nutritional objectives and stay in good health. These tasty parsnip fries are going to become a staple in your culinary arsenal, whether they're served as an appetizer, side dish, or healthy snack. As you enjoy the taste, fragrance, and crispness of these wonderful fries, remember that you are providing your body with nutritious food that has been prepared with care. Celebrate the ease and enjoyment of plant-based eating.

Crunch Edamame with Wasabi

Wasabi Edamame Crunch is a flavorful and wholesome snack that mixes the bold tastes of edamame with a dash of heat from wasabi spice. In addition to being tasty, this crispy, high-protein treat also perfectly fits the low-histamine, vegan diet. Come learn about this tasty snack's advantages and how it may help you achieve your nutritional objectives:

What's in Wasabi Edamame Crunch

- Two cups of frozen peas (shelled)
- 1 tablespoon avocado or olive oil
- A couple of teaspoons of wasabi seasoning (taste-test)
- Add salt to taste, if desired.

Guides

1. Preheat the Oven:
To make cleaning easier, preheat your oven to 400°F (200°C) and line a baking sheet with parchment paper.

2. Get the Edamame Ready:

After freezing, rinse the edamame under cold water to thaw them. To get rid of extra moisture, pat dry with a paper towel.

3. Sprinkle with Oil and Spice:
Toss the thawed edamame with avocado or olive oil in a mixing dish until well coated. Stir in the wasabi seasoning and salt (if used), adjusting the spice to the desired level of heat.

4. Spread on Baking Sheet:
Arrange the seasoned edamame on the baking sheet in a single layer, taking care not to pack them too tightly. This makes roasting and crispiness more uniform.

5. Oven Roasting:
Roast the edamame for 20 to 25 minutes, tossing halfway through, or until they are crispy and browned.

6. Keep Calm and Savor:
Let cool slightly before serving the roasted Wasabi Edamame Crunch. After transferring to a serving dish, enjoy this tasty appetizer or snack.

Healthy Advantages

Edamamé:
Young soybeans, or edamame, are a nutrient-dense legume that is low in histamine and high in fiber, plant-based protein, and minerals like iron and magnesium. It is also high in vitamins like vitamin K and folate. In addition to supporting muscle development and repair, edamame increases satiety and offers vital nutrients for general health.

Sasabi Spice:

Instead of using high-histamine components like standard spicy sauces, wasabi seasoning gives the edamame crunch a distinct and fiery taste. Wasabi is a plant produced from the Japanese horseradish plant that has chemicals that may have antibacterial and anti-inflammatory effects.

Avocado or Olive Oil:
Roasting edamame in avocado or olive oil releases heart-healthy monounsaturated fats and antioxidants while also making the vegetable crispier. These oils add to the snack's overall taste and texture and are appropriate for a low-histamine diet.

Grazing Conscientiously

In addition to being a tasty treat, eating Wasabi Edamame Crunch is a thoughtful decision that promotes your well-being. You may eat this tasty snack by itself, as an accompaniment to salads or grain bowls, or as a delightful treat with your preferred dipping sauce. Enjoy the fiery crunch of Wasabi Edamame Crunch and celebrate the ease and healthfulness of plant-based eating while supporting a bright and well-balanced lifestyle by providing your body with nutrient-rich foods.

Pickled Watermelon Rind

This is a novel and delicious approach to avoiding food waste while enjoying a crunchy, sweet, and tangy snack or condiment. Let's investigate pickled watermelon rinds. I'm thrilled to discuss this handmade treat's health advantages and how it fits within a low-histamine, vegan diet. Come along with me as we go over the specifics of this easy-to-make yet tasty recipe:

Watermelon Rind Pickling Ingredients

- One medium-sized watermelon; Peeled, chopped into bite-sized chunks the rinsed off
- One cup of apple cider vinegar and one cup of water
- Half a cup of granulated sugar or your preferred sweetness
- One tablespoon of salt
- Additives (such as red pepper flakes, cloves, peppercorns, or cinnamon sticks)

Guides

1. Ready the Watermelon Rind:
A medium-sized watermelon should have its outer green skin peeled off without destroying the white rind. Peel the rind and cut it into thin strips or slices, being careful to remove any pink flesh.

2. Construct the Pickling Liquid:
Put the apple cider vinegar, water, salt, sugar (or sweetener), and any other spices in a pot. Stirring periodically, bring the mixture to a boil over medium-high heat until the salt and sugar are completely dissolved.

3. Incorporate the Watermelon Rind:
Place the prepared watermelon rind pieces into the pickling liquid that is boiling. The rind pieces should be soft but still somewhat crunchy after 10 to 15 minutes of simmering over low heat.

4. Keep Cold and Store:
After taking the pot from the stove, let the pickled watermelon rind to come to room temperature. Pour the mixture—including the pickling liquid—into sterile, well-washed jars or other containers.

5. Keep Cold and Savor:
Before serving, be sure to carefully seal the jars or containers and store the pickled watermelon rind in the refrigerator for at least 24 hours. To get the best flavor, pickle the rind for a few days. The tastes will intensify with time.

Healthy Advantages

Red watermelon:
Though it is sometimes disregarded, the rind of watermelon is very nutrient-dense, including minerals like potassium and magnesium, vitamins like C and B vitamins, and antioxidants like lycopene. The skin of the watermelon is preserved with these nutrients and becomes a tasty, crunchy snack or condiment when pickled.

Citrus Distilled Water:
In addition to adding tang, apple cider vinegar to the pickling liquid improves intestinal health and digestion. Known for its possible antibacterial qualities, apple cider vinegar may help control blood sugar levels and encourage weight reduction.

Pickled Watermelon Rind is a great snack right out of the jar, or it can be used as a spicy garnish for tacos, salads, or sandwiches. It may even be served with vegan cheese or charcuterie. Accept the challenge of cutting down on food waste and turning commonplace products into a unique and tasty condiment that will liven up your meals with a hint of sweetness and tang. A tasty and nutritious addition to your vegan low-histamine repertoire, pickled watermelon rinds may be eaten on their own or combined with other ingredients to create delicious dishes.

CHAPTER 8: DELECTABLE DESSERTS

Lavender-infused Blueberry Cheesecake Bites

Dessert lovers, prepare to be enchanted with Lavender-infused Blueberry Cheesecake Bites. For those who suffer from histamine sensitivity, indulging in these mouthwatering sweets is a sin-free pleasure since they not only provide a sensory symphony but also adhere precisely to the guidelines of a low histamine diet. So, let's get down to brass tacks and see how this meal satisfies and nourishes even those with food sensitivities:

Ingredients

- One cup of blueberries, either fresh or frozen
- One tablespoon of culinary lavender buds
- One cup of raw cashews, soaked in water overnight
- A quarter cup of coconut cream
- Two tablespoons of melted coconut oil
- One tablespoon of lemon juice
- A quarter cup of maple syrup or sweetener of choice
- Salt, a pinch
- Vanilla essence, a teaspoon
- For the crust, you may optionally use graham cracker crumbs or crushed nuts.

Its Benefits for Low Histamine Levels

Blueberries:
Blueberries are a low histamine fruit, making them a great option for persons with histamine sensitivity. They are rich in antioxidants, especially flavonoids like anthocyanins, which have anti-inflammatory qualities and may help lower histamine levels in the body.

Culinary Lavender:
Lavender lends a subtle flowery perfume and taste to these cheesecake bites without adding excessive histamine levels. Culinary lavender is recognized for its relaxing qualities and may help ease tension and promote relaxation, helping general well-being.

Raw Cashews:
Cashews serve as the creamy foundation for the cheesecake filling and are good for a low histamine diet when ingested in their raw form. They contain healthy fats, protein, and critical elements like magnesium and zinc, boosting energy generation and immunological function.

Coconut Cream:
Coconut cream offers richness and creaminess to the cheesecake filling without possessing excessive histamine levels. It is a dairy-free alternative to regular cream cheese and offers a mild coconut taste that compliments the blueberries and lavender well.

Instructions for Preparation

1. Prepare the Blueberry-Lavender Compote:
Simmer fresh or frozen blueberries with culinary lavender buds until they release their juices and make a fragrant

compote. Let it cool before using it as a tasty topping for the cheesecake bites.

2. Make the Cheesecake Filling:
Blend soaking raw cashews with coconut cream, maple syrup, melted coconut oil, lemon juice, vanilla essence, and a bit of salt until smooth and creamy. This delectable filling serves as the ideal canvas for the blueberry-lavender compote.

3. Assemble and Chill:
Layer the cheesecake mixture over a graham cracker crust or crushed nuts in tiny muffin cups or silicone molds. Top with the chilled blueberry-lavender compote and refrigerate in the refrigerator until hard.

4. Garnish and Serve:
Before serving, top the Lavender-infused Blueberry Cheesecake Bites with fresh blueberries, lavender blossoms, or a drizzle of maple syrup for extra sweetness and visual appeal.

As you enjoy these Lavender-infused Blueberry Cheesecake Bites, take time to appreciate the harmonious balance of tastes and the nutritional benefits they give. Each mouthful is a celebration of culinary ingenuity and thoughtful eating, delivering a delicious retreat while accommodating your dietary requirements and preferences. Share these scrumptious delicacies with loved ones and indulge in the thrill of appreciating life's little pleasures, one mouthful at a time.

Saffron and Cardamom Rice Pudding

Prepare to go on a gastronomic adventure via the magical tastes of Saffron and Cardamom Rice Pudding—a timeless delicacy adored in cultures throughout the globe for its creamy texture and fragrant spices. I wish to convey the joys of this wonderful dessert and how it may be enjoyed as part of a balanced and healthy diet. Let's delve into the specifics and study the rich history, nutritional advantages, and preparation of this luscious treat:

History and Cultural Significance

Rice pudding has a long and storied history, extending back centuries and spanning numerous countries and cuisines. Known by many names such as kheer in India, arroz con leche in Latin America, and riz au lait in France, rice pudding maintains a distinct position in culinary traditions worldwide. The addition of saffron and cardamom infuses this traditional dessert with the exotic aromas of the Middle East and South Asia, producing a sensory experience that thrills the tongue and inspires memories of other locations.

Ingredients for Saffron and Cardamom Rice Pudding

- 1/2 cup basmati rice
- 4 cups whole milk or coconut milk for a dairy-free alternative
- 1/2 cup sugar or sweetener of choice
- 1/4 teaspoon saffron threads
- 4-5 green cardamom pods, gently smashed

- 1/4 cup chopped nuts (such as almonds, pistachios, or cashews) for garnish (optional)
- Dried rose petals for garnish (optional)

Nutritional Benefits

Basmati Rice:
Basmati rice is a long-grain rice type recognized for its fragrant scent and fluffy texture. It is naturally gluten-free and low in histamine, making it acceptable for persons with food sensitivities. Basmati rice delivers complex carbs for sustained energy, as well as tiny levels of protein and fiber.

Saffron:
Saffron is a treasured spice originating from the crocus flower and appreciated for its brilliant color and unusual taste. It includes antioxidants such as crocin and crocetin, which may have anti-inflammatory and mood-enhancing qualities. Saffron gives a rich touch to the rice pudding and boosts its visual attractiveness.

Cardamom:
Cardamom is a fragrant spice with warm, lemony undertones that enhance the richness of the rice pudding. It includes chemicals including cineole and terpinene, which may improve digestion and support general gut health. Cardamom is also high in antioxidants and has been utilized in traditional medicine for its possible health benefits.

Instructions for Preparation

1. Rinse and Soak the Rice:

Rinse the basmati rice under cold water until the water runs clear. Soak the rice in water for 30 minutes to 1 hour to soften the grains and shorten the cooking time.

2. Infuse the Milk:
In a heavy-bottomed saucepan, boil the whole milk or coconut milk over medium heat until it comes to a moderate simmer. Add the saffron threads and crushed cardamom pods to the milk, allowing them to absorb their flavors into the liquid.

3. Cook the Rice:
Drain the soaked rice and add it to the boiling milk mixture. Stirring periodically, cook the rice over medium-low heat until it becomes soft and absorbs most of the liquid. This procedure may take 30-40 minutes, depending on the desired consistency of the pudding.

4. Sweeten and Flavor:
Once the rice is cooked to your taste, add sugar or sweetener of choice to the pudding, stirring until it is entirely dissolved. Adjust the sweetness according to your desire. You may also add a dash of rose water or vanilla essence for added taste.

5. Serve and Garnish:
Remove the cardamom pods from the rice pudding and discard them. Transfer the pudding to serving dishes or glasses and decorate with chopped nuts and dried rose petals for a touch of elegance and texture. Serve the saffron and cardamom rice pudding warm or cold, according to your liking.

As you delight in the creamy richness of Saffron & Cardamom Rice Pudding, take a minute to absorb the subtle tastes and smells that dance on your palette. The gentle sweetness of the rice pudding, combined with the exotic flavors of saffron and cardamom, takes you to other regions and produces a feeling of warmth and comfort. Whether savored as a warm dessert after a meal or as a sumptuous treat for special occasions, this timeless classic promises to satisfy your senses and feed your spirit with every mouthful. Embrace the history and culinary legacy of rice pudding as you build treasured memories and moments of delight with loved ones, one exquisite mouthful at a time.

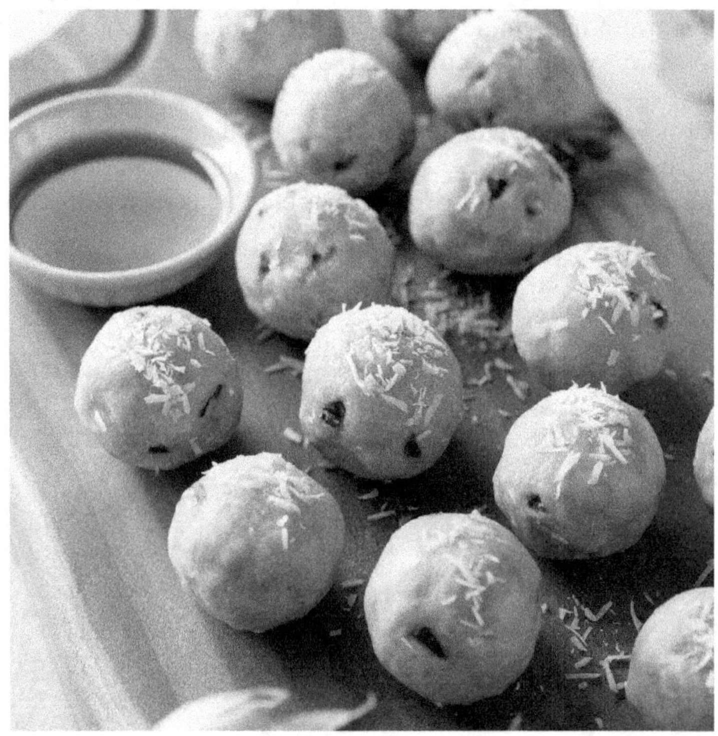

Embark on a voyage of taste and energy with Pistachio Rosewater Energy Balls—a delectable snack that mixes the earthy richness of pistachios with the delicate floral tones of rosewater. Allow me to introduce you to this delicious delicacy that not only fulfills your desires but also delivers a surge of energy and nutrients to support your busy lifestyle. Let's delve into the specifics and find the compelling allure of these nutritious energy balls:

Ingredients for Pistachio Rosewater Energy Balls

- 1 cup shelled pistachios
- 1 cup pitted dates, steeped in warm water for 10-15 minutes
- 1 tablespoon rosewater
- 1/4 cup shredded coconut (optional, for coating)
- 1-2 teaspoons water, as required

Nutritional Benefits

Pistachios:
Pistachios are nutrient-dense nuts rich in healthy fats, protein, fiber, and key elements including vitamin E, potassium, and magnesium. They give prolonged energy and increase satiety, making them a perfect element for energy balls. Pistachios are particularly low in histamine, making them ideal for persons with food sensitivities.

Dates:
Dates act as a natural sweetener and binder in these energy balls, offering a strong supply of carbs for rapid energy. They are abundant in fiber, antioxidants, and minerals including potassium and magnesium, supporting digestive health and muscular function.

Rosewater:
Rosewater provides a gentle floral perfume and taste to the energy balls, improving their sensory appeal and delivering a refreshing twist. Rosewater is generated from rose petals and includes chemicals including flavonoids and polyphenols, which may have antioxidant and anti-inflammatory effects.

Instructions for Preparation

1. Prepare the Ingredients:
In a food processor, pulse the shelled pistachios until finely chopped, but not powdered. Drain the soaked dates and put them in the food processor along with the chopped pistachios and rosewater.

2. Blend Until Smooth:
Blend the mixture until it creates a sticky dough-like consistency, adding 1-2 teaspoons of water as required to help bind the ingredients together. The dough should keep its form when squeezed between your fingers.

3. Shape Into Balls:
Using your hands, shape the dough into tiny balls, approximately 1 inch in diameter. If preferred, roll the energy balls in shredded coconut for extra texture and taste.

4. Chill and Set:
Place the formed energy balls on a baking sheet coated with parchment paper and refrigerate for at least 30 minutes to let them firm up and solidify. This helps the balls keep their form and makes them simpler to handle.

5. Serve and Enjoy:
Once cooled, transfer the Pistachio Rosewater Energy Balls to an airtight container and keep them in the refrigerator for up to one week. Enjoy them as a handy snack on the move, a pre-workout boost, or a sweet treat to satiate your desires.

As you sample the Pistachio Rosewater Energy Balls, experience the perfect combination of tastes and textures that stimulate your senses and energize your taste receptors. The creamy richness of pistachios, coupled with the gentle sweetness of dates and the delicate scent of rosewater, produces a symphony of flavor that thrills the palette and feeds the body. Whether consumed as a noon pick-me-up or a post-workout refill, these nutritious energy balls give a quick and tasty way to feed your day with natural goodness and vigor. Embrace the delight of snacking mindfully as you indulge in these healthy snacks, knowing that you are feeding your body and spirit with every mouthful.

CHAPTER 9: BEVERAGES TO REFRESH AND REJUVENATE

Cooling Lemongrass and Ginger Iced Tea

Prepare to quench your thirst and energize your senses with Cooling Lemongrass and Ginger Iced Tea—a reviving beverage that mixes the delicious scents of lemongrass and ginger with the coolness of iced tea. Let's get into the specifics and investigate the calming characteristics and nutritional benefits of this revitalizing drink:

Ingredients for Cooling Lemongrass and Ginger Iced Tea

- 4 cups water
- 2 stalks of lemongrass, cut and smashed
- A 1-inch piece of fresh ginger, sliced
- 2-3 tablespoons honey or sweetener of choice (optional)
- Juice of 1-2 lemons or limes
- Ice cubes
- Fresh lemongrass stalks and ginger slices for garnish (optional)

Nutritional Benefits

Lemongrass:

Lemongrass is appreciated for its pleasant citrus taste and fragrant characteristics. It includes essential oils including citral and limonene, which have antioxidant and anti-inflammatory qualities. Lemongrass is also rich in vitamins A and C, boosting immune function and skin health.

Ginger:
Ginger lends a fiery bite and warmth to the iced tea, making it both stimulating and calming. Gingerol, the main ingredient in ginger, has significant anti-inflammatory and digestive benefits. Ginger is also recognized for its ability to reduce nausea and enhance circulation.

Instructions for Preparation

1. Infuse the Water:
In a saucepan, bring the water to a boil over medium heat. Add the crushed lemongrass stalks and sliced ginger to the boiling water, allowing them to absorb their flavors into the liquid. Reduce the heat to low and simmer for 10-15 minutes.

2. Sweeten to Taste:
If desired, sweeten the infused tea with honey or your choice sweetener, swirling until dissolved. Adjust the sweetness according to your liking, keeping in mind that the acidity of the lemon juice will also provide a natural sweetness to the tea.

3. Add Citrus Juice:
Remove the pot from the heat and mix in the freshly squeezed lemon or lime juice. The citrus juice lends a tangy brightness to the iced tea, boosting its taste profile and offering a dose of vitamin C.

4. Chill and Strain:
Allow the infused tea to cool to room temperature before filtering it through a fine-mesh strainer to remove the lemongrass stalks and ginger slices. Transfer the filtered tea to a pitcher and refrigerate until cooled.

5. Serve Over Ice:
Fill glasses with ice cubes and pour the cooled Lemongrass and Ginger Iced Tea over the ice. Garnish each glass with a fresh lemongrass stalk or ginger slice for an exquisite touch and additional scent.

As you sip on Cooling Lemongrass & Ginger Iced Tea, let the refreshing tastes and stimulating scents take you to a state of serenity and relaxation. This refreshing beverage not only hydrates the body but also comforts the spirit, offering a moment of relief from the rush and bustle of everyday life. Whether savored as a lunchtime refreshment, a post-workout cooldown, or a calming bedtime treat, Lemongrass and Ginger Iced Tea provide a lovely way to refresh and restore your senses while feeding your body with natural goodness. Embrace the simple joys of sipping on a nice glass of iced tea and cherish the moment as you indulge in this hydrating elixir, knowing that you are prioritizing your health and well-being with every sip.

Matcha Mint Mojito Smoothie

Prepare to raise your beverage game with the Matcha Mint Mojito Smoothie—a vivid and invigorating combination that blends the antioxidant-rich richness of matcha with the refreshing zest of mint and lime.

Ingredients for Matcha Mint Mojito Smoothie

- 1 cup unsweetened almond milk or coconut milk
- 1 tablespoon matcha powder
- 1 ripe banana, frozen
- Handful of fresh mint leaves
- Juice of 1 lime
- 1-2 tablespoons honey or sweetener of choice (optional)
- Ice cubes

Nutritional Benefits

Matcha Powder:
Matcha is a finely powdered powder created from green tea leaves, recognized for its high antioxidant benefits and beautiful green color. It contains catechins, especially epigallocatechin gallate (EGCG), which have been associated with many health advantages, including increased brain function, enhanced metabolism, and lower risk of chronic illnesses.

Mint:
Mint offers a refreshing blast of flavor to the smoothie, waking the senses and delivering a cooling feeling. It includes menthol, which has been proven to reduce intestinal pain and induce relaxation. Mint is also rich in vitamins and minerals, including vitamin A, vitamin C, and manganese.

Instructions for Preparation

1. Blend the Ingredients:
In a blender, add the unsweetened almond milk or coconut milk, matcha powder, frozen banana, fresh mint leaves, lime juice, and honey or sweetener of choice, if using. Blend until smooth and creamy, adjusting the sweetness and consistency to your suit.

2. Add Ice Cubes:
For an added refreshing touch, add a handful of ice cubes to the blender and process again until the smoothie achieves your chosen degree of frostiness. The ice cubes help cool the smoothie and provide a slushy texture that is excellent for hot summer days or post-workout refreshments.

3. Garnish and Serve:
Pour the Matcha Mint Mojito Smoothie into glasses and decorate each drink with a sprig of fresh mint or a slice of lime for a flash of color and extra scent. Serve immediately and enjoy the stimulating taste of this refreshing beverage.

As you take a drink of the Matcha Mint Mojito Smoothie, let the vivid tastes and fragrant scent transport you to a state of renewal and energy. This delightful combination of matcha, mint, and lime wakes your senses and invigorates your taste buds, offering a surge of energy and nutrients to power your day. Whether consumed as a morning pick-me-up, a noon refresher, or a post-workout recovery drink, the Matcha Mint Mojito Smoothie is a delicious way to invigorate your body and mind with every sip. Embrace the simple pleasure of sipping on this vivid green elixir and cherish the moment as you indulge in the benefits of matcha and mint, knowing that you are prioritizing your health and well-being with every delightful sip.

Ingredients for Hibiscus and Orange Blossom Elixir

- 4 cups water
- 1/2 cup dried hibiscus blossoms
- Zest of 1 orange
- Juice of 2 oranges
- 2 tablespoons honey or sweetener of choice (optional)
- 1-2 tablespoons orange blossom water
- Ice cubes
- Orange slices and fresh mint leaves for garnish (optional)

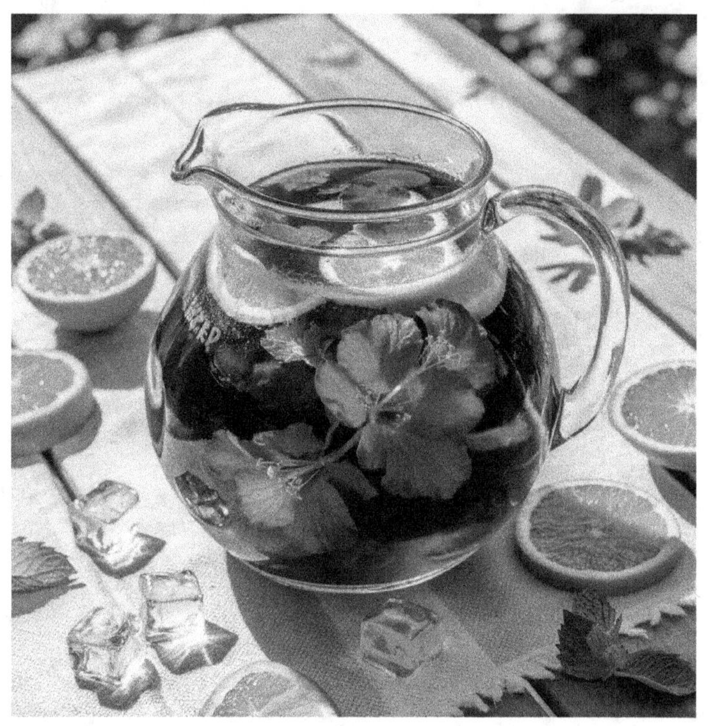

Nutritional Benefits

Hibiscus Flowers:
Hibiscus is a tropical flower noted for its brilliant red color and acidic taste. It is rich in antioxidants, particularly flavonoids, and anthocyanins, which have been found to decrease blood pressure, enhance cholesterol levels, and promote heart health. Hibiscus also contains anti-inflammatory qualities and may assist with digestion.

Orange Zest and Juice:

Oranges are a significant source of vitamin C, a potent antioxidant that promotes immunological function and collagen formation. The zest and juice of oranges lend a blast of zesty flavor to the elixir, increasing its scent and delivering a refreshing tanginess. Oranges also include fiber, potassium, and other critical elements that enhance general health and well-being.

Instructions for Preparation

1. Infuse the Water:
In a saucepan, bring the water to a boil over medium heat. Add the dried hibiscus flowers and orange zest to the boiling water, swirling gently to immerse the ingredients. Reduce the heat to low and simmer for 10-15 minutes to allow the flavors to mingle.

2. Sweeten to Taste:
Once the hibiscus mixture has simmered, take it from the heat and filter off the hibiscus flowers and orange zest using a fine-mesh strainer or cheesecloth. Stir in honey or sweetener of choice, if preferred, until well dissolved.

3. Add Citrus and Floral Notes:
Allow the hibiscus-infused liquid to cool slightly before whisking in the freshly squeezed orange juice and orange blossom water. The orange juice offers a vibrant zesty taste, while the orange blossom water contributes a beautiful flowery scent to the elixir.

4. Chill and Serve:
Transfer the Hibiscus and Orange Blossom Elixir to a pitcher and refrigerate until well cold. When ready to serve, pour the elixir into glasses filled with ice cubes and garnish each glass

with an orange slice and a sprig of fresh mint for a touch of elegance.

As you sip on the Hibiscus and Orange Blossom Elixir, let the brilliant colors and aromatic smells take you to a state of relaxation and renewal. This delightful elixir not only quenches your thirst but also feeds your body with a surge of antioxidants and vitamins. Whether sipped as a morning refresher, a noon pick-me-up, or a calming bedtime treat, the Hibiscus and Orange Blossom Elixir is a pleasant way to fill your day with natural goodness and vigor. Embrace the simple pleasure of sipping on this vivid elixir and cherish the moment as you indulge in its refreshing aromas and nutritious characteristics, knowing that you are prioritizing your health and well-being with every sip.

CHAPTER 10

Tips for Dining Out and Socializing - Navigating
Menus with Confidence

Embark on a voyage of culinary discovery with confidence as you peruse menus and mingle while following your vegan low-histamine diet. Dining out and enjoying social events may be enjoyable experiences packed with varied cuisines and discussions. As a professional nutritionist, I'm here to give informative suggestions to help you make educated decisions and relish the moment without sacrificing your dietary preferences or health objectives. Let's go into the art of browsing menus with confidence and grace:

Plan Ahead

Before going out to a restaurant or social gathering, take a proactive approach by reviewing the establishment's menu online. Many restaurants now provide thorough menus or allergy information on their websites, enabling you to select vegan and low-histamine alternatives in advance. Consider phoning the restaurant ahead of time to ask about food substitutions or modifications.

Communicate Clearly

When eating out, don't hesitate to mention your dietary preferences and limits to the waitress or chef. Politely ask inquiries regarding menu items, including how they are created and if particular components may be deleted or swapped. Most eateries are friendly and prepared to alter meals to match your demands.

Focus on Whole Foods

Opt for recipes that feature entire, unprocessed components such as vegetables, legumes, grains, and plant-based proteins. Choose salads, roasted vegetable platters, grain bowls, or vegetable-based curries that are naturally low in histamine and rich in nutrients. Avoid foods that are severely processed, cured, or fermented, since they may contain greater amounts of histamine.

Be Mindful of Seasonings and Sauces

Histamine levels might fluctuate based on the flavors and sauces used in restaurant food. Be wary of foods that are seasoned with fermented condiments like soy sauce, fish sauce, or vinegar-based sauces. Instead, prefer basic spices like olive oil, lemon juice, fresh herbs, or non-histamine alternatives.

Choose Fresh and Light Options

Opt for lighter meals that are less prone to induce histamine responses. Fresh salads, grilled veggies, steamed meals, and simple stir-fries are wonderful alternatives. Avoid deep-fried meals, aged cheeses, processed meats, and sweets with high sugar content, since they may increase histamine intolerance symptoms.

Stay Hydrated

Drink lots of water during your eating experience to keep hydrated and help digestion. Avoid alcoholic beverages, carbonated drinks, and caffeinated beverages, since they might stimulate histamine release or increase symptoms of intolerance.

Enjoy the Experience

Remember that eating out is not just about sustenance but also fun and social interaction. Focus on the presence of friends or loved ones, participate in meaningful discussions, and eat each mouthful attentively. Embrace the chance to experience new tastes and culinary creations that suit your nutritional choices.

Be Flexible and Patient

Keep in mind that eating out while following a vegan low-histamine diet may need flexibility and patience. Not every restaurant will offer clear alternatives on the menu, but most are ready to accommodate dietary demands with a little imagination. Approach each eating experience with an open mind and a pleasant attitude.

By following these ideas and principles, you may peruse menus with confidence and elegance while enjoying the delights of eating out and mingling. Embrace the variety of culinary experiences, fight for your dietary choices, and relish the delight of shared meals with others. With smart preparation and communication, you can make eating out a rewarding and pleasurable aspect of your lifestyle while emphasizing your health and well-being.

Sharing Your Dietary Needs with Friends and Family

Embrace the adventure of communicating your dietary preferences with friends and family as you navigate social events and eating experiences. Communicating your choices and constraints with loved ones may build understanding, support, and meaningful relationships. I'm here to give insight on how to approach these talks with clarity, compassion, and confidence. Let's examine techniques for communicating your dietary preferences with friends and family in a manner that promotes connections and enriches your eating experiences:

Choose the Right Moment

Find a safe and calm location to discuss your dietary requirements with friends and family. Avoid bringing up the matter around mealtimes or when emotions are high. Instead, find a moment when everyone is calm and amenable to open conversation.

Explain Your Reasons

Be candid about the reasons behind your dietary choices or limits. Share information on your vegan low histamine diet, including how it promotes your health and well-being. Educate your friends and family about histamine intolerance and the necessity of treating symptoms via food adjustments.

Emphasize Inclusivity

Assure your friends and family that your food choices are not meant to bother or disturb their plans. Express thanks for their willingness to accommodate your demands and reassure them that you are devoted to finding solutions that work for everyone. Emphasize the value of inclusion and finding common ground in shared experiences.

Offer Solutions

Propose practical ideas or alternatives that make it simpler for friends and family to satisfy your dietary demands. Suggest arranging potluck-style parties so everyone may offer foods that match their dietary choices. Offer to share recipes or item ideas to make meal preparation easier.

Be Patient and Understanding

Recognize that not everyone may completely understand or instantly appreciate your dietary choices. Be patient and empathetic in your relationships, providing friends and family members time to adjust and adapt to your demands. Encourage open discussion and be responsive to questions or concerns they may have.

Lead by Example

Lead by example and highlight the wonderful and rewarding alternatives accessible within your vegan low-histamine diet. Prepare delectable foods to share with friends and family, showing that eating healthfully can be pleasurable and gratifying. Encourage trial and exploration of new foods and cuisines together.

Focus on Connection

Above all, value the connection and camaraderie enjoyed with friends and family at meals and gatherings. Emphasize the satisfaction of spending quality time together, participating in meaningful discussions, and making enduring memories. Celebrate the link that food develops and the shared experiences that bring people together.

By addressing talks about your dietary preferences with care and understanding, you may develop stronger ties with friends and family while navigating social occasions with confidence and grace. Embrace the chance to teach and inspire people about the advantages of a vegan low histamine diet, and develop a supportive community that supports diversity and inclusiveness. Together, you may enjoy the delights of shared meals and create memorable moments that nurture both body and spirit.

CONCLUSION

As we conclude our journey, let us reflect on the inspiring adventure of adopting a vibrant vegan histamine lifestyle. Throughout this book, we've studied the subtle balance between sustenance, health, and gourmet enjoyment, empowering you to take charge of your dietary choices and enhance your well-being. Now, let's weave together the strands of knowledge, experience, and inspiration into a tapestry of change and life.

Honoring Your Body

At the core of a thriving vegan low histamine diet is a profound regard for the body's intrinsic knowledge and resilience. By listening to your body's signals and recognizing its unique requirements, you start on a path of self-discovery and self-care. Embrace the power of healthy meals, mindful exercise, and restorative activities that support your body's natural healing processes and promote overall vitality.

Cultivating Awareness

In the quest for good health, information is your best ally. Cultivate awareness of the meals you eat, the substances they contain, and the influence they have on your body. By understanding the concepts of histamine intolerance and the role of nutrition in treating symptoms, you get the ability to make educated decisions that correspond with your health objectives and beliefs.

Celebrating Diversity

Embrace the wonderful tapestry of tastes, textures, and smells that the vegan low-histamine diet has to offer. Celebrate the variety of plant-based products and culinary traditions from across the globe, infusing your meals with creativity, passion, and pleasure. Let each mouthful be a celebration of life, replenishing not just your body but also your soul.

Nurturing Connection

Food is more than simply nutrition; it is a powerful vehicle for connection, community, and celebration. Share your journey with others, encouraging friends and family to join you in enjoying the pleasures of vegan low-histamine cooking. Cultivate genuine friendships through shared meals, sincere talks, and acts of kindness that feed the spirit as much as they do the body.

Embracing Balance

In the search for health and vigor, remember the need for balance and moderation. Embrace the 80/20 rule, giving yourself the freedom to enjoy occasional indulgences while keeping a foundation of healthful, balanced meals. Listen to your body's instincts, practice intuitive eating, and recognize its desire for variety, pleasure, and nutrition.

Seizing the Moment

As you begin on this road of adopting a vibrant vegan low histamine lifestyle, grab each moment with appreciation and purpose. Embrace the beauty of the current moment, relishing the tastes, feelings, and experiences that enhance your life. Let each meal be a mindful meditation, a time of rest and introspection in a fast-paced society.

Inspiring Change

As you embrace the ideas of a lively vegan low histamine lifestyle, you become a light of inspiration and transformation in your own life and the lives of others. Share your expertise, experiences, and recipes with compassion and kindness, enabling others to begin on their path of health and well-being.

In conclusion, may you continue to appreciate the diverse tapestry of tastes, sensations, and experiences that the vegan low-histamine lifestyle has to offer. May you feed your body, nurture your spirit, and build relationships that improve your life and the world around you. Remember, the road toward optimum health is not a destination but a constant evolution—a voyage of self-discovery, development, and change. Embrace it with open arms and an open heart, knowing that you can create a life of energy, joy, and plenty.

BONUS

One-Week Meal Plan

Day 1

Breakfast: Energizing Dragon Fruit Smoothie Bowl
Lunch: Creamy Kohlrabi Soup with Lemongrass
Dinner: Spicy Eggplant and Peanut Stew
Snack: Wasabi Edamame Crunch
Dessert: Lavender-infused Blueberry Cheesecake Bites
Beverage: Cooling Lemongrass and Ginger Iced Tea

Day 2

Breakfast: Coconut Milk Porridge with Cardamom and Saffron
Lunch: Tangy Jicama Salad with Tamarind Dressing
Dinner: Roasted Beetroot and Orange Salad with Pistachio Vinaigrette
Snack: Crispy Baked Parsnip Fries with Rosemary Salt
Dessert: Saffron and Cardamom Rice Pudding
Beverage: Hibiscus and Orange Blossom Elixir

Day 3

Breakfast: Golden Turmeric Breakfast Muffins
Lunch: Creamy Kohlrabi Soup with Lemongrass (leftovers)
Dinner: Tempeh Kebabs with Pineapple Salsa
Snack: Matcha Mint Mojito Smoothie

Dessert: Pistachio Rosewater Energy Balls

Day 4

Breakfast: Lavender-infused Blueberry Cheesecake Bites
Lunch: Tangy Jicama Salad with Tamarind Dressing (leftovers)
Dinner: Saffron and Cardamom Rice Pudding
Snack: Wasabi Edamame Crunch
Dessert: Coconut Milk Porridge with Cardamom and Saffron
Beverage: Cooling Lemongrass and Ginger Iced Tea

Day 5

Breakfast: Coconut Milk Porridge with Cardamom and Saffron
Lunch: Creamy Kohlrabi Soup with Lemongrass (leftovers)
Dinner: Crispy Baked Parsnip Fries with Rosemary Salt
Dessert: Lavender-infused Blueberry Cheesecake Bites

Day 6

Breakfast: Golden Turmeric Breakfast Muffins
Lunch: Tangy Jicama Salad with Tamarind Dressing
Dinner: Tempeh Kebabs with Pineapple Salsa
Snack: Crispy Baked Parsnip Fries with Rosemary Salt
Dessert: Saffron and Cardamom Rice Pudding
Beverage: Hibiscus and Orange Blossom Elixir

Day 7

Breakfast: Energizing Dragon Fruit Smoothie Bowl
Lunch: Creamy Kohlrabi Soup with Lemongrass
Dinner: Spicy Eggplant and Peanut Stew

Snack: Matcha Mint Mojito Smoothie
Dessert: Pistachio Rosewater Energy Balls

This one-week meal plan offers a variety of flavorful and nutritious dishes for breakfast, lunch, and dinner, as well as satisfying snacks, desserts, and beverages. Enjoy the diverse array of flavors and textures while nourishing your body and supporting your health and well-being. Cheers to delicious and wholesome eating!

Additional Recipes

Here are some other recipes along with preparation instructions:

Hot Szechuan Stir-Fried Eggplant

Ingredients include:

- 2 big eggplants, diced
- 2 tablespoons soy sauce
- 1 tablespoon rice vinegar
- 1 tablespoon maple syrup
- 1 tablespoon sesame oil
- 2 minced garlic cloves
- 1 teaspoon grated ginger
- 1 tablespoon crushed
- Szechuan peppercorns
- 2 sliced green onions.
- Ready-to-serve cooked rice

Guidelines:

1. In a big pan or wok over medium heat, warm up one tablespoon of sesame oil.
2. Add the diced eggplant to the pan and simmer for 5 to 7 minutes or until tender.
3. Combine the soy sauce, grated ginger, rice vinegar, maple syrup, and chopped garlic in a small bowl.
4. After adding the sauce to the cooked eggplant, toss everything together.
5. Stir-fry the crushed Szechuan peppercorns in the pan for an additional two to three minutes.
6. Add sliced green onions as a garnish and serve hot over cooked rice. Savor the fragrant and spicy stir-fried Szechuan eggplant!

Tofu Glazed with Miso and Gingered Greens

Ingredients include:

- One block of firm tofu that has been pressed and cut into rectangles
- Two teaspoons of white miso paste
- Two tablespoons of maple syrup
- One tablespoon each of rice vinegar and soy sauce.
- 1-Tbsp sesame oil
- Garlic (2 cloves)
- 1 tablespoon grated ginger
- 4 cups mixed greens (bok choy, spinach, or kale, for example)
- As a garnish, toast sesame seeds

Guidelines:

1. Turn the oven on to 400°F, or 200°C. Put parchment paper on one side of a baking sheet.

2. To prepare the glaze, combine the white miso paste, grated ginger, pine nuts, rice vinegar, soy sauce, chopped garlic, and sesame oil in a small dish.

3. Arrange the tofu slices on the baking sheet that has been prepped, then drizzle with the miso glaze on both sides.

4. Bake the tofu in the oven for 20 to 25 minutes, or until crispy and golden brown.

5. Meanwhile, get the greens ready (ginger, spinach). In a big skillet over medium heat, preheat one tablespoon of sesame oil.

6. Put the mixed greens in the pan and cook them for three to five minutes, or until they wilt.

7. Present the warm miso-glazed tofu with mixed greens, topped with toasted sesame seeds. Savor the spicy and sweet elements of this delectable meal!

Quinoa Pilaf with Herbed Stuffed Portobello Mushrooms

Ingredients:

- 1 cup rinsed and drained quinoa
- 2 cups vegetable broth
- 1 tablespoon olive oil
- 1 small onion, chopped
- 2 minced cloves of garlic
- One teaspoon each of dried thyme and rosemary
- One-fourth cup of finely chopped fresh parsley
- Salt and pepper to taste

Guidelines:

1. Set the oven's temperature to 375°F or 190°C. Put parchment paper on one side of a baking sheet.
2. Place the gill-side-up portobello mushrooms on the baking sheet that has been prepped.
3. Heat the vegetable broth in a medium saucepan until it begins to boil. When the quinoa is soft and the liquid has been absorbed, add the rinsed quinoa, lower the heat to low, and simmer covered for 15 to 20 minutes.
4. Meanwhile, bring a pan of olive oil to medium heat. Saute the minced garlic and chopped onion until they become tender.
5. Cook for a further minute after adding the dried thyme and rosemary.
6. After the quinoa is cooked, use a fork to fluff it up and move it into a mixing dish. Mix well to include the chopped parsley, salt, and pepper, as well as the sautéed onion and garlic combination.
7. Gently push the quinoa pilaf into the inside of each portobello mushroom by spooning it in and packing it in.
8. Bake the filled portobello mushrooms in the preheated oven for twenty to twenty-five minutes, or until the quinoa is lightly brown and the mushrooms are soft.
9. Garnish the heated-filled portobello mushrooms with more fresh parsley, if preferred. Savor the rich and savory fusion of herbed quinoa pilaf with mushrooms!

These additional dishes will stimulate your culinary imagination and satiate your palate with a range of tastes and textures. Savor the effort of preparing these delectable dishes and the knowledge that every mouthful is a celebration of healthful ingredients and creative cookery.